The Impact of Inequality

"Richard Wilkinson's pathbreaking work challenges everyone interested in socio-economic conditions and health to rethink in a most constructive way. This new book brings insight into how conditions of society impact on people's daily lives to cause health and disease. It is a stimulating and exciting book." *Professor Sir Michael Marmot, Professor of Epidemiology and Public Health, Royal Free and University College Medical School, London.*

"Wilkinson's work is a powerful and provocative piece of scholarship. *The Impact of Inequality* presents a challenge to us all to improve population health by tackling economic and social inequalities." *Lisa Berkman, Thomas D. Cabot Professor of Public Policy, Harvard School of Public Health.*

Why do people in more unequal societies have worse health and shorter lives? And why are levels of violence higher and community life weaker where there is more inequality?

In this book, pioneering social epidemiologist Richard Wilkinson shows how inequality affects social relations and gets under people's skin. In wealthy countries, health is not simply a matter of material circumstances and access to health care; it is also how your relationships and social standing make you feel about life.

Using detailed evidence from rich market democracies, *The Impact of Inequality* addresses people's experience of inequality and presents a radical theory of the psychosocial impact of class stratification. The book demonstrates how poor health, high rates of violence and low levels of social capital all reflect the stresses of inequality. It also explains the pervasive sense that, despite material success, our societies are sometimes social failures. What emerges is a new conception of what it means to say that we are social beings and of how the social structure penetrates our personal lives and relationships.

Richard G. Wilkinson's careful analysis of a vast field of fascinating research shows that we should not wait to reach an unattainable level of equality, and leaves us in no doubt that even small reductions in inequality matter. The book ends by outlining the political and economic changes required to improve wellbeing and the quality of life for us all.

Richard G. Wilkinson is Professor of Social Epidemiology, Division of Epidemiology and Public Health, University of Nottingham Medical School, and Visiting Professor at the International Centre for Health and Society, Department of Epidemiology, University College London. He has been researching the social determinants of health and health inequalities for over 25 years and is the author of the bestselling *Unhealthy Societies: The Afflictions of Inequality* (Routledge, 1996).

health studies/health policy/medical sociology

The Impact of Inequality

How to make sick societies healthier

RICHARD G. WILKINSON

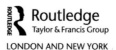
Routledge
Taylor & Francis Group

LONDON AND NEW YORK

First published in the UK in 2005 by Routledge
2 Park Square, Milton Park, Abingdon,
Oxfordshire, OX14 4RN
Tel: +44 020 7017 6000
Fax: +44 020 7017 6699

Reprinted 2006 (three times)

Routledge is an imprint of the Taylor & Francis Group, an informa business

Published in the USA in 2005 by The New Press, New York

© 2005 Richard G. Wilkinson

Printed and bound in Great Britain by TJ International Ltd,
Padstow, Cornwall

Every effort has been made to ensure that the advice and information in
this book are true and accurate at the time of going to press. However,
neither the publisher nor the authors can accept any legal responsibility
or liability for any errors or omissions that may be made. In the case of
drug administration, any medical procedure or the use of technical
equipment mentioned within this book, you are strongly advised to
consult the manufacturer's guidelines.

British Library Cataloguing in Publication Data
A catalogue record for this book is available from the British Library

ISBN10: 0-415-37268-2 (hbk)
ISBN10: 0-415-37269-0 (pbk)

ISBN13: 978-0-415-37268-8 (hbk)
ISBN13: 978-0-415-37269-5 (pbk)

Contents

Preface

As this book is primarily a work of synthesis, I am indebted to a large number of people whose work has provided the pieces of the jigsaw puzzle I have attempted to fit together. Although there have been numerous discussions and some arguments about how they fit together, what has struck me throughout the thirty years I have been thinking about these issues is people's profound sense of commitment to their work, to its social purposes, and to concepts of social justice that have motivated the long hours of painstaking research work. Rarely, if ever, have disagreements been about trivial or unworthy issues. As a result, and despite usually working alone. I have felt part of a wider community bound together not only by a commitment to research on health inequalities and the determinants of health and well-being in the population but also by the issues of social justice they raise. I therefore feel a deep sense of gratitude to a network of supportive friends and colleagues, and to a few whose interpretations have made them formidable rivals.

Despite the danger that such a long list of names will lead to an expectation that it will end "and Uncle Tom Cobbley and all," I would like to express my special thanks to the following for the way they have—in different combinations—affected my thinking, set admirably high standards in research, shown me kindness and support, and done the research on which I draw: Mel Bartley, Lisa Berkman, Stephen Bezruchka, David Blane, Mildred Blaxter, Martin Bobak, Eric Brunner, Simon Charlesworth, Helena Cronin, George Davey Smith, Angus Deaton, David Donnison, Danny Dorling, Jim Dunn, David Erdal, Sarah Fan, Luisa Franzini, Paul Gilbert, Pam Gillies, David Halpern, Clyde Hertzman, Ichiro Kawachi, Shona Kelly, Bruce Kennedy, Margareta Kristenson, Barbara Krimgold, Di Kuh, Anton Kunst, Peter Lobmayer, David Lowe, Johan Mackenbach, Michael Marmot, Sally McIntyre, Kate Pickett, Chris Power, Pauline

Rosenau, Nancy Ross, Robert Sapolsky, Mary Shaw, Aubrey Sheiham, Carol Shively, Johannes Siegrist, Alvin Tarlov, Roberto de Vogli, Mike Wadsworth, Patrick West, David Williams, Michael Wolfson, and Alison Ziller. The world would be a poorer place without them and the contributions they have made to the development of a new field that brings the benefit of scientific investigation to bear on one of the key issues of social justice facing modern societies.

Over the years I have been supported financially by both the Economic and Social Research Council and the Medical Research Council in Britain, by several charities—including the Baring Foundation and the Paul Hamlyn Foundation—and, most recently, by the University of Nottingham. Without the university's (and my departmental colleagues') forbearance, I would never have completed this volume.

1
Affluent Societies
Material Success, Social Failure

Within each of the developed countries, including the United States, average life expectancy is five, ten, or even fifteen years shorter for people living in the poorest areas compared to those in the richest. This huge loss of life, reflecting the very different social and economic circumstances in which people live, stands as a stark abuse of human rights. Although we tend to assume that class differences have been diminishing in modern societies, during the last few decades the health differences between classes have increased. They reveal such a gulf between the lives and experience of rich and poor, well educated and less well educated, and, through the same social and economic stratification, different racial or ethnic groups, that they call into question the humanity, morality, and values of modern societies.

This book is not a guide to the dos and don'ts of healthy behavior. Instead, it uses the research on these health differences to explore the effects social and economic inequality have on us as individuals and on whole societies. An understanding of such gross effects of social stratification takes us to a deeper understanding of the societies we live in. Because health standards are most powerfully determined by social factors, it takes us to the roots of the social malaise affecting many of the richest societies and suggests the kind of changes that are likely to increase not only the length of life but, much more importantly, the subjective social quality of life for all of us.

With the provision of sewers and clean water supplies, the public health movement of the nineteenth century led to a transformation of the physical environment in our cities. Our growing understanding of the social determinants of health in modern societies has the potential to usher in another, more fundamental transformation in the quality of our lives. By identifying what it is about the social structure that does the damage, we initiate a program of reform that will allow future generations, with the benefit of hindsight, to see how disfigured our societies and social relations really were.

Changing Lifetimes

A family photo taken almost ninety years ago shows my mother as a baby sitting on her grandmother's knee. My mother, now also age ninety, is still alive; her grandmother, on whose knee she was sitting, was born in 1826. (In case that sounds as if it stretches the time limits on female reproductive capability, I should point out that the connection between them is through my mother's *father*.) Eighteen twenty-six was three years before Stephenson's "Rocket," the primitive steam engine that, pulling a load at thirteen miles an hour, won its historic victory by demonstrating the potential of mechanical over animal power. These two overlapping lives stretch from the dawn of mechanical power to a world in which air travel has shrunk what were once long and dangerous voyages by sail to a few hours; they stretch from before the first integrated national postal service to modern global electronic communications. They also stretch over equally large social and political changes: from when slavery was still widespread and public executions and floggings were common even for minor crimes to the present, when in all the more progressive developed countries (including all members of the European Union but excluding the United States) all forms of corporal and capital punishment are banned, and teachers and sometimes even parents are not allowed to slap children.

Despite the extraordinary speed of change, the economic growth rates that drove so much of this forward would now be regarded as little better than stagnation. Throughout the world's first industrial revolution, which took place in Britain, economic growth rates rarely exceeded 1 percent a year. Growth rates now have to be at least three times that to be regarded as respectable, and a few countries grow ten times as fast. Remarkable though the extraordinary transformations of the recent past are, the pace of change is accelerating.

To match this, our thinking has to be radical. From a time when it took a generation or two for what was beyond imagination to become reality, we now find that what was unthinkable in our early adulthood becomes reality before the end of our lives. This means that we have to think ahead on the grand scale, grasping the essential dynamics of the forces that are driving our society forward, asking not only where they are taking us but where we want to go, what we can do to avoid the worst pitfalls, and how we can steer our societies toward happier outcomes.

So advanced are modern living standards that we have almost forgotten what extraordinary luxuries basics such as running hot water and good sewage systems would have seemed to our ancestors. It is difficult to recognize the difference made by even such simple innovations as window glass, common for only the last few centuries, which achieves the near magical combination of letting light into our homes while keeping cold winds out. And now, in the developed countries, even the poor have washing machines, vacuum cleaners, refrigerator-freezers, TVs, VCRs, and often cars.

Yet these same societies often seem deeply unhappy places, coping with a heavy burden of depression, anxiety, stress, and dependency on psychoactive drugs—including alcohol and illegal and prescribed drugs—not to mention high crime rates. Despite unprecedented material comfort, luxury, and safety, we nevertheless use a vocabulary of stress and survival as if it sometimes seemed almost impossibly difficult just to keep going. Although work is physically easier and working hours are shorter, stress is the most common cause of sickness-related absences. Psychosocial problems are the single most common reason for consulting a doctor, and the largest group of drug prescriptions are for psychoactive drugs or painkillers to help us cope with depression, anxiety, sleeplessness, and so on. They calm us down, reduce pain, and often stimulate pleasure centers in the brain as well. Everywhere a substantial minority of people are close to the edge of breakdown, feeling their endurance and ability to cope stretched to the limit, close to giving up the struggle to continue, vulnerable to paranoia, likely to be isolated and living alone, and sometimes even prey to bizarre and occasionally dangerous fantasies. Even over the last half century, when we can base judgments on similar standards, the best evidence suggests that in most countries depression has actually become more common (rather than just more widely recognized), suicide rates have risen, alcoholism has increased, and crime rates are higher.

The contrast between the material success and social failure of modern societies is a profound paradox, and we have little understanding of the causal processes responsible for it. Our predecessors would have expected us to revel in the extraordinary ease produced by seemingly miraculous technology, which not only keeps us in material plenty while at the same time replacing most of the hard grind of muscle power with machines, but tops it off with so many dizzying luxuries we now take for granted, such as the perfectly reproduced sound of a symphony orchestra in our homes or cars at the touch of a button, the ability to watch events as they happen on the other side of the world, or the possibility of talking to anyone, anywhere, from wherever we happen to be.

Most of our predecessors would have predicted that material prosperity would usher in an extraordinary flourishing of social life: meanness and animosity would ebb as human sociality was liberated from the divisive effects of scarcity. In an affluent world, surely social life would become marked by an unstinted human warmth and generosity. But the social development of our societies provides little to boast about. It certainly falls a very long way short of inspiring the pride and confidence to match what we might feel about many of the achievements of modern science and technology.

Many of our predecessors regarded scarcity as the root of a great deal of social conflict. Even the hard-nosed seventeenth-century political thinker Thomas Hobbes believed that competition for scarce resources was unquestionably the most important source of human conflict. But for the overriding power of a monarch or government capable of enforcing peace, Hobbes believed that competition for scarce resources threatened to reduce society to the "warre of each against all."

On the other side of the political spectrum, early socialists made similar assumptions about the effects of scarcity. They thought the state of plenty that industrialization seemed to be bringing would establish new political and economic systems and usher in an era of human brother- and sisterhood, free of class divisions and war.

So what has gone wrong? Why do we so often feel miserable, stressed, and near desperation—as if the extraordinary physical comfort, the plethora of entertainment and opportunities for every kind of interest and stimulation, meant nothing?

From time to time commentators suggest that our problems spring from the way affluence has weakened the force of necessity in our lives: in effect, our liberation brings our downfall with it. Necessity, the guiding principle in our lives for generations, suddenly loosens its grip on us and leaves us with a debilitating freedom. If this were true, the problems would be most severe in the richest sections of society, where people are most liberated from necessity. But there is endless statistical evidence showing that almost every social problem and sign of unhappiness is more common (usually much more common) in the poorest areas and sections of society, exactly where the force of necessity remains strongest.

Measures of social well-being used to increase in parallel with wealth as countries got richer during the course of economic development. But now, although rich countries have continued to get richer, measures of well-being have ceased to rise, and some have even fallen back a little. Since the 1970s or earlier, there has been no increase in average well-being despite rapid increases in wealth.

With few exceptions, remarkably little real effort or well-informed debate is devoted to trying to understand why prosperity has not brought the social benefits that might have been expected of it. Too often politicians and media commentators prefer to play to public prejudices rather than heed the evidence we have. And most of us, as private individuals, are more likely to join the rising tide of consumerism in an attempt to keep our spirits up—insofar as our overextended credit limits allow. For the more seriously disaffected, binge drinking and drugs often seem to offer the best chance of finding, however briefly, the social and emotional ease we crave.

As a society, however, we are enormously much better placed than ever before to develop some kind of understanding of our condition and what is going wrong. Carefully used, computers and statistical analyses provide us with something like a social microscope, revealing relationships we either failed to see or preferred to deny. As a result, we can now begin to understand the social processes in which we are enmeshed. As humanity becomes more aware of its position in the universe—the age of our planet, the evolution of our species, how our minds and bodies work—we are also becoming more aware that to understand ourselves we need to understand the societies we are part of. In a bumbling, self-serving, or self-justifying kind of way, the social sciences provide modern societies with their own self-awareness or self-consciousness. As this becomes less partial—less bound to the interests of just one class, one religion, one race, or one country, above all others—the more moralistic and reactionary views, which have often led to entirely counterproductive responses to social problems, are giving way to a more unified view of our humanity and what it means to be human.

Health as a Social Indicator

Much of the evidence we will be looking at to see how we are affected by different aspects of the societies in which we live comes from studies originally undertaken to identify some of the main influences on health and longevity in the developed countries. Over the last two decades or so, research on what have come to be called the "social determinants of health" has been a major source of new insights into the way we are affected by our social environment and the social structures in which we live.

Health and illness reflect the nature of the interface between ourselves and the environment. The fact that most, if not all, diseases have some environmental cause means that their initiation, or the course of the disease process, is an expression of the interaction between us and our surroundings. Diseases arise at the friction points in our relationship with the environment: they show when our circumstances get the better of us, just as good health shows that things are working satisfactorily for us. The illnesses we get may be seen as telling us what is going wrong in that interaction. Whether an individual suffers from depression, the effects of alcoholism, ulcers, heart disease, obesity, anxiety disorders, lung disease, or some kind of cancer, a knowledge of the causes of these conditions usually tells us what aspects of someone's life are going wrong.

Using health as a kind of social indicator provides important social and psychological insights. It is revealing because different conditions reflect what is going on in quite different areas of life. Although many diseases are affected primarily by material conditions, what makes this a particularly exciting field is that many others are powerfully affected by, and therefore indicative of, our choice of lifestyle and our social and emotional well-being.

Recent research has revealed that some intensely social factors are among the most important determinants of health in the rich countries. These include the nature of early childhood experience, the amount of anxiety and worry we suffer, the quality of our social relationships, the amount of control we have over our lives, and our social status. By choosing which dimensions of health we look at and what angle we look at them from, we can choose what aspects of life health tells us about.

If, on top of that, we look not just at the health of individuals but at data for whole societies or at differences between groups within the population, the chanciness of individual situations balances out to reveal wider and more reliable patterns and relationships.

The Epidemiological Transition

Social and psychological factors loom large among the determinants of health in the developed countries because the long history of rising living standards has drastically reduced the direct effects of material privation. The impact of increasing incomes and the decline of absolute poverty stand out very clearly in the health record. "The epidemiological transition" is the name given to the changes in health brought about by economic development as it lifted populations out of absolute material want.

The most important feature of the epidemiological transition is the well-known process by which the old infectious causes of death, which killed people at all ages but particularly in childhood, gave way to degenerative diseases such as cardiovascular diseases and cancers, which appear mainly in later life. While the old infectious diseases still remain the diseases of poverty in the third world today, the degenerative diseases of old age have become the main causes of death in the developed countries.

Health in societies that have gone through the epidemiological transition ceases to be as responsive to further rises in material living standards as it had been earlier. Once you have enough of everything, it doesn't help to have much more. Once the important material preconditions for health have been established, the curve of rising life expectancy with increasing gross national product (GNP) per capita levels off. Hence, life expectancy among the twenty-five or thirty richest countries is no longer related to how rich they are. For example, although the United States is much the richest country in the world and spends very much more than any other on medical care, life expectancy in the United States is shorter than it is in most other developed countries—including some that are only half as rich. Even among the fifty U.S. states there is little or no relation between average income and life expectancy. Although the population in some states is twice as rich as others, there is no tendency for that to be reflected in differences in average longevity (Wilkinson 1997a).

Another particularly interesting feature of the epidemiological transition shows even more clearly that we are now beyond the point at which a substantial proportion of the population has to worry about access to basic necessities in the way they once did. As infectious diseases declined, many of the so-called diseases of affluence reversed their social class distribution to become more common among the poor in affluent societies. For example, heart disease, which had been a rich man's disease more common in the upper classes, became a disease of the poor in affluent countries. The same thing happened with a number of other conditions, including stroke and lung cancer. Most indicative of all perhaps is the reversal in the social distribution of obesity. For centuries the rich have been fat and the poor have been thin, but when we came out of the epidemiological transition the pattern reversed and the tendency became, as it is now, for the poor to be fatter than the rich.

When, in the first half of the twentieth century, heart disease was still a rich man's disease, poverty was still defined in terms of absolute material want. However, soon after the middle of the twentieth century, higher wages and living standards, supported by various welfare safety nets, had rescued most people from the threat of the worst forms of deprivation. And just as the rich countries came out of the epidemiological transition and obesity and heart disease became more common lower down the social scale, poverty began to be redefined in relative rather than absolute terms. Now even official poverty lines in European Union countries (though not in the United States) are defined in relative rather than absolute terms (typically as living on less than half the national average income), and poverty's impact is redefined in terms of "social exclusion."

Rather like the way receding floodwaters reveal the nature of the underlying terrain, so the influence of psychosocial factors on health has become increasingly visible as the force of material privation has declined. But it was not only the fact that they were hidden by the powerful direct effects of material poverty that made psychosocial factors difficult to see in poorer countries. It was also because absolute material want is itself a source of great worry and anxiety, so material deprivation and psychological stress were almost inseparable. Shortages of food or of other basic material necessities would always be accompanied by the effects of psychological and social stress. Another factor tending to hide the power of psychosocial influences on health is that stress affects health partly by increasing people's vulnerability to other pathogens. So, for instance, because experiencing prolonged stress downregulates our bodies' immune systems, it makes us more vulnerable to whatever infections we may be exposed to. The result, again, is that instead of appearing independently, the health effects of stress often operate in conjunction with exposure to sources of infection.

The biology of how psychosocial factors affect health seems to hinge predominantly on the extent to which they cause frequent or recurrent stress. Chronic stress affects numerous physiological systems, including the cardiovascular and immune systems, increasing our vulnerability to a very wide range of diseases and health conditions. So widespread are its effects that we should perhaps think of it as a general vulnerability factor whose effects may be analogous to more rapid aging. Although there are a number of more subtle physiological indicators, psychosocial influences on health show up in the rich countries most obviously in health-related behavior (such as smoking, drinking, drug abuse, and eating "for comfort") and in the earlier onset of the degenerative conditions of later life.

What makes health a really important social indicator is that psychosocial risk factors for disease reflect how we think, feel, experience, and suffer our lives. Understanding them means understanding the social meanings of people's circumstances. Psychosocial risk factors for poor health are particularly informative when it comes to understanding the social malaise in many of the rich market democracies because the main sources of stress are so closely intertwined with the widespread signs of unhappiness in modern societies. Because psychosocial factors influence health through stress, the main psychosocial risk factors identified by research are also likely to be the most important sources and symptoms of chronic stress in modern societies. They include depression, anxiety, helplessness, hostility, isolation, insecurity, and lack of a sense of control—not to mention the pressures that lead people to dependency on prescribed or recreational drugs (including tobacco and alcohol). Not only do all of these exert powerful influences on health and on death rates, but their prevalence is central to the sense that social improvements have failed to keep up with the technological achievements of the modern world.

In short, it is because the various forms of psychological pain and misery make such an important addition to the burden of physical disease and shortening of life that health research provides such a powerful way of understanding the social failure of modern societies. On the positive side, feeling happy and in control of life, having friends, and enjoying good relationships all seem highly beneficial to health.

Perhaps unsurprisingly, it is to the nature of the social environment and social relationships that we have to look to identify the most powerful causes of stress in modern life. And although the social environment of any particular individual may seem entirely fortuitous, reflecting only chance effects in personal circumstance, epidemiological studies of health—sometimes collecting data from many thousands of people—show some remarkably reliable patterns that help us relate the psychosocial well-being of the population to features of the social structure.

Health Inequalities

Where these issues come most sharply into focus is in research designed to understand the causes of health inequalities—the large social class differences in health and life expectancy that disfigure modern societies, which we mentioned at the start of this chapter. Within societies, health is graded by social status. Whether we look at life expectancy or at the frequency of most causes of death and disability, health standards are highest among those nearest the top of the social ladder—whether measured by income, education, or occupation—and lower as we look at each successive step down the ladder.

Research (Geronimus et al. 2001) using official data from twenty-three rich and poor areas in the United States found that white women who had reached the age of sixteen and were living in the richest areas could expect to live until they were eighty-six years old, compared to seventy for black women in the poorest areas of New York, Chicago, and Los Angeles—a difference of sixteen years. Similarly, sixteen-year-old white men living in rich areas could expect to live until they were seventy-four or seventy-five, whereas black men in the poorest areas could expect to live to only about fifty-nine. The difference in life expectancy between whites in rich areas and blacks in poor areas of the United States was close to sixteen years for both men and women. If the figures had been for life expectancy *at birth,* so taking into account deaths in infancy and childhood, the life expectancy gap would have been even larger. Death rates in all twenty-three areas were very closely related to median household income in each area, and differences in area incomes almost wholly accounted for differences in black and white death rates. This means that in the United States, health inequalities related to differences in socioeconomic circumstances may involve depriving the average person in the poorest communities of as much as 20 percent—or, if we take life expectancy at birth, perhaps more like 25 percent—of the length of life that people in the richest communities enjoy. As a result, the poorest areas of the United States, such as Harlem in New York or the South Side of Chicago, have death rates that are higher at most ages than in Bangladesh—one of the poorest countries in the world (McCord and Freeman 1990).

But this is not simply about extremes of wealth and poverty. There is a continuous gradient in death rates all the way through society—even among the middle classes. The higher people's status, the longer they live. A follow-up study of seventeen thousand men working in government offices in London found that death rates from heart disease were four times as high among the most junior office workers as among the most senior administrators working in the same offices (Rose and Marmot 1981). Intermediate levels in the office hierarchy had intermediate death rates. Most of the differences could not be explained by the most well-known risk factors for heart disease, including the behavioral ones, such as smoking, exercise, and diet, which explained less than one-third of the health differences in this and other studies (Lantz et al. 1998). Nor are these health differences due to just one or two diseases: most causes of death tend to be more common lower down the social hierarchy, and rather few are more common among the better-off. When looking at deaths from all causes combined, rather than just from heart disease, the same study of government office workers in London found that death rates were three times as high among the junior employees as among the senior staff. (Throughout this book, all comparisons of death rates are adjusted for differences in the age and sex composition of the populations being compared.) These huge health disparities occur among office workers who would mostly call themselves "middle class." If the poor, the unemployed, and the homeless had been included, the health differences would have been substantially larger.

Rather than being simply a problem of poverty, the health gradient runs through all classes from top to bottom of society to the extent that, even if we managed to remove all the health problems associated with poverty, the greater part of health inequalities would remain untouched. Even the health chances of readers of this book, and their chances of having a long and healthy retirement, are graded by socioeconomic status.

A crucially important point to recognize about health inequalities is that the scale of health differences varies from society to society and from one period to the next. For instance, countries such as the United States, and more recently Britain, have larger health differences than most of the social democratic European countries—particularly the Nordic countries. Table 1 shows how the health gap has changed in Britain during recent decades. It compares differences in life expectancy between people in professional occupations (social class I) and people in unskilled manual occupations (social class V) in England and Wales. In the early 1970s men and women in social class V jobs had lives that were about five and a half years shorter than those of men and women in social class I. By the early or mid-1990s, these differences had increased dramatically, to nine and a half years for men and nearly six and a half years for women. After that, there appears to have been at least some decline in the differences, but the gap was still substantially bigger than it had been in the early 1970s. Although the disadvantage of class V decreased, there was little or no sign of a general reduction in the steepness of the class gradient in life expectancy across the intermediate classes. That there are differences in health inequalities from one country to another and from one period to the next shows that they should not be regarded as fixed or inevitable. It suggests that they can be very substantially reduced.

Table 1.1

Changes in occupational class differences in life expectancy at birth (England and Wales)

	Occupational class I (professional occupations) compared to Occupational class V (unskilled manual occupations)	
	Male	**Female**
1972–76	5.5 years	5.3 years
1992–96	9.5 years	6.4 years
1997–99	7.4 years	5.7 years

Source: A. Donkin, P. Goldblatt, and K. Lynch, "Inequalities in Life Expectancy by Social Class 1972–1999," *Health Statistics Quarterly* 52 (2002):15–19.

Such large differences in life expectancy represent the most serious social injustices scarring modern market democracies, whatever their causes. We are used to feeling indignation at the human rights abuses in countries where people are imprisoned without trial, are tortured, or simply disappear, but health inequalities exact a much greater toll. What would we think of a ruthless government that arbitrarily imprisoned all less well-off people for a number of years equal to the average shortening of life suffered by the less privileged in our own societies? Given that higher death rates are more like arbitrary execution than imprisonment, perhaps we should liken the injustice of health inequalities to that of a government that executed a significant proportion of its population each year without cause.

The higher death rates suffered by people lower down the social hierarchy are, however, only half the injustice. The other half is that life is short where its quality is poor: the health injustice reflects another underlying injustice. If lives were shortened primarily because people ate too many french fries or doughnuts, we could at least say their lives were short and sweet. But an important part of the reason for the shortening of life involves forms of social and psychological stress, including depression and anxiety, that dominate people's whole experience of life.

As well as being a fundamental issue of social justice, health inequalities also provide an epidemiological clue to the most important determinants of health standards in populations. Fortunately, there has been a substantial, publicly funded, international research effort focused on understanding health inequalities. Though many issues are highly contested, and government decisions to fund research may often be an alternative to taking effective political action, it is rare for an empirical problem that so profoundly reflects social injustice to receive concerted scientific attention.

The evidence on which this book is based comes from a very large number of research findings. Some studies have used prospective methods, following many thousands of people over decades, sometimes from birth; included as well are cross-sectional, individual, and area studies. Difficulties in distinguishing between correlation and causality that could not be settled using follow-up studies have sometimes been overcome by evidence from intervention studies, so-called natural experiments, and occasionally studies of other primate species. Although this evidence points to deep-seated problems in our societies, it cannot be shrugged off or ignored.

Some of the most powerful factors contributing to the social gradient in health have turned out to be very different from what many of us engaged in this research would initially have guessed; indeed, the importance of psychosocial factors was unexpected. But in addition to the surprises about what society has to tell us about health, health has also told us an unexpectedly interesting story about society. It has provided new kinds of evidence and a new vantage point from which to view some of the most challenging social and political issues facing rich societies. In particular, it has told us more about the relationship between the individual and society and how we are affected by social structures.

In understanding the causes of health inequalities we are, to a substantial extent, also casting light on important causes of a wide variety of other social problems. It is not just that they share poor health's association with relative deprivation and low social status: they also share many of the same psychosocial pathways. Social problems—such as violence, drug use, depression, teenage pregnancy, and poor educational performance of schoolchildren—are rooted in the same insecurities, anxieties, and other sources of chronic stress as those that affect our ability to withstand disease, the functioning of our cardiovascular and immune systems, and how rapidly we age.

This concentration on psychosocial processes does not mean that the problems of material life are ignored—rather the opposite. Because social structures and the quality of social relations in society at large are, as we shall see, built on material foundations (so that the characteristics of social and material relations run parallel to each other), this book is centrally concerned with understanding the effects of socio-economic and income inequalities on the nature of social life. There are still people who say that greater material inequality does not matter, who think that only the absolute levels of income and wealth enjoyed by a society matter. That is a view that can no longer be sustained in the face of the evidence.

As well as looking at how inequality affects death rates, the quality of social relations, levels of violence, and involvement in community life, we shall also find out what it is about us, as human beings, that explains why inequality is so socially corrosive. As we get a better understanding of the sources of these problems, we come to understand our social nature and some of the features of society that would improve well-being and the quality of life.

But this book is not a moral diatribe against inequality. It is an attempt to show the empirical evidence of the social effects of inequality and to develop an explanation of them.

The explanation takes us to the evolutionary roots of human sociality. Still, although it is an empirical analysis, the resulting picture does of course have moral implications, not only because of the effects of inequality on those at the bottom, but also for what it does to the social fabric of society. The analysis and conclusions have strong implications for the desirable future direction of social change in our societies.

Another reason this book is not simply a diatribe against inequality or an expression of some unrealistic utopian ideal of perfect equality is that the evidence comes almost entirely from statistical comparisons of the effects of the different amounts of inequality found among the developed market economies today. Although it may well be better to be more egalitarian than any of these countries are today, what the statistical evidence shows is that even the existing small differences in the levels of inequality in different societies matter. They have important implications for the quality of life of all of us.

Summary and Plan of Chapters

The core argument in this book is that to understand the benefits of greater equality we need to understand our responses to inequality and dominance hierarchies, and that means understanding the social life of monkeys at least as much as it means understanding the writings of political theorists of class such as Marx.

At the most fundamental level we, like other species, have to solve the fundamental problem of competition for scarce resources. Because members of the same species have the same needs, there is always a huge potential for conflict over access to the necessities of life. There are two contrasting ways of dealing with the potential for conflict, and the extent of inequality is a fairly good indicator of where we are on the spectrum between them. At one extreme are the dominance hierarchies, based on power and coercion, in which the lion's share goes to the strongest and social relations are ordered according to differentials in power as a reflection of the potential for conflict. At the other extreme is the egalitarian solution, based on fairness and a recognition of each other's needs. The adoption of this solution among our prehistoric hunting and gathering ancestors explains the predominance of reciprocity, gift exchange, and food sharing in early human societies. The contrast is between relationships based on power and fear and those based on social obligations, equality, and cooperation. The extent of inequality in any society tells us a lot about where on this continuum the society lies.

Appropriate to each pattern of social relationship we have deeply ingrained matching social strategies that equip us either for dominance relationships, in which other people are feared rivals, the strong prey on the weak, everyone tries to gain advantage in the social hierarchy, and people exploit each other when they can, or for affiliative relationships, in which other people are the best source of mutual aid, friendship, cooperation, and security. Given that so much is at stake, and that the best social strategies to use are so different in each context, we have necessarily become highly attentive to the nature of social relations: timid or fearful in the presence of superiors, and at ease and secure among friends.

But what is exciting is that, as we shall see demonstrated empirically, the balance between the social strategies seems to be powerfully triggered by differences in the degree of equality or inequality in our social environment. Inequality promotes strategies that are more self-interested, less affiliative, often highly antisocial, more stressful, and likely to give rise to higher levels of violence, poorer community relations, and worse health. In contrast, the less unequal societies tend to be much more affiliative, less violent, more supportive and inclusive, and marked by better health. It looks almost as if human nature could be developed to produce nearly any mix—from people bordering on antisocial personalities with limited powers of empathy and little sense of responsibility for the common good to the opposite. The extent of dominance hierarchies and the social strategies we adopt also have a powerful influence on whom we find sexually attractive and on reproductive strategies more widely.

Figure 1.1: The effects of income inequality (left-hand side) on social and psychological well-being (right-hand side)

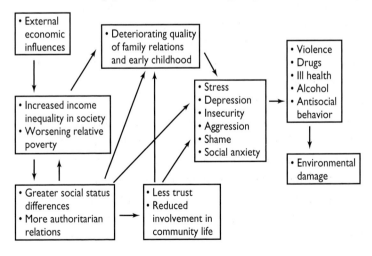

Social processes cannot be reduced to box diagrams with arrows to show the direction of the causal links, but figure 1.1 is an attempt to do just that. At least, the words in the different boxes serve to flag the range of issues discussed in the coming chapters. As everything in the social world affects everything else, every box in the diagram could be linked with bidirectional arrows to every other. The figure is an attempt to suggest the causal processes that lead from greater material inequality, on the left-hand side, to various psychological, behavioral, and health outcomes, on the right. The arrows indicate the stronger social processes discussed in this book.

The subsequent chapters fall into two groups: chapters 2, 3, and 4 outline research findings that provide a picture of the basic relationships indicating how inequality affects us and the societies we live in. The remaining chapters explain the causal processes which account for these relationships. So we start off seeing what is affected by the amount of inequality in a society and then go on to see how and why inequality has these effects.

Following this introductory chapter, chapter 2 presents evidence showing that the quality of social relations in societies is related to the scale of income inequality—how big the gap is between rich and poor. It shows that more unequal societies tend to have higher rates of violent crime and homicide, and that people living in them feel more hostility, are less likely to be involved in community life, and are much less likely to trust each other; in short, they have lower levels of social capital. The data in this chapter show just how deeply corrosive inequality is.

Chapter 3 shifts the focus from the quality of social relations at the societal level to the main individual psychosocial risk factors leading to ill health and premature death. Because psychosocial factors affect health through the extent to which they trigger biological stress responses, what the epidemiological research on psychosocial risk factors has done amounts to nothing less than the identification of the most important sources of stress in modern societies. It is the power of psychosocial risk factors for health, rooted as they are in chronic stress, that explains why health research provides such an important new vantage point from which to understand the problems of modern societies. Most important are three intensely social risk factors. First is low social status, which in this context is less a matter of low material living standards themselves than of their social consequences, such as feeling looked down on, having an inferior position in the social hierarchy, and subordination (and therefore also a reduced ability to control one's circumstances and work). Second comes poor social affiliations of all kinds, including lack of friends, being single, weak social networks, lack of involvement in community life, and so on. Under the auspices of social status and social affiliations come the contrasting social strategies and the extent to which they are brought into play in different social environments. Third comes early childhood experience, which prepares us to deal with more conflict-ridden or more affiliative social environments. It includes pre- and postnatal stress, both of which have lifelong effects on stress and health. The effects of maternal stress in pregnancy on fetal development combine with the effects of stress in early childhood—associated with things such as poor attachment or domestic conflict—to program, or "tune," stress responses during a continuous period of early sensitivity to stress stretching from before birth into childhood.

Everyone needs to feel valued and respected, have friends, and have had the advantage of an early childhood that provides the basis for self-confidence in adult life. But in addition to these apparently personal and individual factors affecting our vulnerability to stress (and to all the health and social problems that arise from it), there are also societal factors that make these issues more problematic in some societies than others. Social status differentials have a huge impact on whether people feel valued, appreciated, and needed or, on the other hand, looked down on, ignored, treated as insignificant, disrespected, stigmatized, and humiliated. And one of the most powerful influences on how important social status differentials are in a society is the scale of income differentials.

In chapter 4 we move on to discuss the evidence that more unequal societies also tend to have higher death rates. Looking at the three categories of psychosocial risk factors discussed in chapter 3, we should expect health to be worse where there are larger income differences. Not only is there a larger burden of relative deprivation lower down in society but, as chapter 2 shows, the quality of social relations also tends to be poorer. In addition, family life is likely to be more stressed for the large number of people who have to cope with the difficulties of living in relative poverty. (This is particularly important in societies where a large proportion of families with children live in relative poverty.) The data showing that more unequal societies tend to have worse health build upon and confirm the material in the previous two chapters. The pathway runs from inequality, through its effects on social relations and the problems of low social status and family functioning, to its impact on stress and health.

We then move on to the second part of the book, which

puts flesh on the bones of earlier chapters and provides a deeper understanding of why inequality has the effects described. Rather than simply showing the evidence that violence, the quality of social relations, and health are all related to inequality, chapter 5 begins to explain the psychological and behavioral processes that lie behind these relationships. Concentrating on violence as a way into understanding what is going on, this chapter shows that the reason violence is more common in more unequal societies is because inequality and the burden of low social status increase the likelihood that people will feel disrespected and looked down on. That violent incidents are so often triggered by loss of face and people feeling they are being "dissed" or looked down on, shows the extent to which inequality and low social status are assaults on our sense of dignity and self-worth. The chapter also looks briefly at how these problems relate to self-esteem.

Taking those themes a step further, chapter 6 describes some of the social processes that help create social distances and distinctions, snobbishness, and the tendency to discriminate against people further down the social hierarchy, all of which become more pronounced where there are bigger income inequalities. It contrasts these dominance strategies with the much more affiliative and cooperative social strategies, appropriate to friendship and social alliances, that are more likely to flourish between equals. It is this contrast, tied to the extent of inequality and social hierarchy, which explains why the quality of social relations is better in more egalitarian societies.

Chapter 6 also discusses the question of which way causality runs in the relationship between inequality and the quality of social relations. Does greater inequality lead to a deterioration in the quality of social relations, or do changes in the quality of social relations lead to changes in income inequality? The discussion looks at a number of examples and pieces of evidence and concludes that although causality can go in either direction, it much more frequently goes from changes in income inequality to changes in the quality of social relations than vice versa.

Chapter 7 continues the discussion in chapter 5 but shows how racism and the status of women in relation to men are affected by dominance strategies. Societies with more inequalities and stronger dominance hierarchies have tended, to the detriment of women, to be more male-dominated or patriarchal. Because more-unequal societies are less sociable, more aggressive, and more violent, the status of women in them is much less likely to improve. In societies where dominance hierarchies are strongly emphasized, there is a tendency found not only among humans but also among a number of other primates for individuals who have been humiliated by a more dominant individual to show what has often been called "displaced aggression" toward weaker or more vulnerable individuals or groups—in effect, to reassert their status and authority over whomever they can. In his analysis of the Nazi scapegoating of the Jews during the Holocaust, Theodor Adorno (Adorno et al. 1950) described this as the "bicycling reaction" because, in authoritarian social structures with strong ranking systems, people bow to their superiors (as if leaning forward on a bicycle) while kicking down on subordinates. The tendency is for societies with bigger inequalities to show more discrimination against vulnerable groups, whether women or religious or ethnic minorities.

Chapter 8 starts by pointing out that human beings have

lived in social systems ranging from the highly egalitarian hunting and gathering societies of human prehistory to the most tyrannical of dictatorships. Such differences in our human and prehuman evolutionary past required quite different social strategies. If you are a baboon living in a dominance hierarchy, you watch your back, keep out of the way of your superiors, and have to be ready to fight for what you can get. But in the more egalitarian societies of human prehistory, people invested in social relations and used gift exchange and food sharing to ensure that they could enjoy the benefits of reciprocity and cooperation. With people so dependent on reciprocity and mutual support, their security was inextricably related to the strength of their social relationships.

In this context chapter 8 has three tasks, all related in different ways to the demands of social life and the way different forms of social organization have etched themselves into human psychology and biology. The first is a discussion of our ingrained responses to more or less egalitarian social environments and why differences in this dimension of social relations matter to us as much as they do—bringing out either more affiliative behavior, or a repertoire of dominance and ranking strategies. The second is to outline how the programming of stress responses in early childhood serves to prepare us for more or less affiliative social structures. The third task is simply to outline some of the biological mechanisms through which the stress associated with dominance hierarchies has health consequences—basically how stress not only affects behavior but gets under the skin to affect our cardiovascular and immune systems.

Finally, chapter 9 starts by pointing out that the picture emerging from this analysis—and indeed from social epidemiology—focuses attention on three crucial dimensions of the social environment that have long been seen as key political objectives: liberty, equality, and fraternity. By liberty the French revolutionaries of 1789 did not mean freedom of consumer choice; they meant not being subservient or beholden to the arbitrary power of the feudal nobility and landed aristocracy. The demand for liberty was fundamentally an attack on social status differentials, closely related to the social costs of dominance hierarchies and low social status. In gender-neutral terms, fraternity refers to the importance of the quality of social relations in modern society, reflected in levels of violence, trust, friendship, and involvement in community life. Equality comes in as the precondition for both liberty and fraternity. Great material inequality not only produces all the problems of low social status—such as people feeling devalued and looked down on—but, as the data and theory suggest, also damages the quality of social relations.

In effect, the main sources of stress and of the psychosocial risk factors for ill health to which research has drawn our attention seem to be just those dimensions of the social environment people have always thought crucial to the real quality of life. However, the costs of our failure to get these things right are not confined to the social or human costs. Greater inequality is perhaps the most significant obstacle to the development of an environmentally sustainable level of economic activity. By increasing status competition, inequality adds to the pressure to consume as a way of expressing social status. It condemns us to ever-spiraling economic growth, destruction of resources, and environmental pollution. Chapter 9 ends by drawing attention to some of the political objectives—including forms of economic and institutional democracy—we need to pursue if we are to improve the psy-chosocial quality of life and stop using consumption as an in-dividualistic, but zero-sum, cure for social ills.

Rather than making do with a vague idea that perhaps in-equality is socially corrosive, it is essential that we should de-velop a more thorough understanding of how we are affected by inequality if we are to make headway in solving the prob-lems of modern societies. And rather than dismissing the rela-tionships that show how we are affected by inequality as utopian, as if they made a difference only if we could achieve some perfect equality, it is important to remember that all the data used in this book come from existing societies, primarily market democracies. This means that there are numerous practical policies that could help heal the sores of modern so-cieties and dramatically improve the quality of life for all of us.

The themes addressed in this book cover a set of tightly in-terlocking social processes. Because the same issues recur, it has been hard to avoid repetition. For instance, levels of vio-lence come up in chapter 2 as one of the indicators of the quality of social relations. They come up again when we look in chapter 5 at people's sensitivity to being put down and treated as inferior. It is also part of the discussion in chapter 7 of discrimination against women and ethnic minorities. Sev-eral other themes are picked up more than once in the book, but repetition has of course been kept to a minimum.

2

Inequality
More Hostile, Less Sociable Societies

The evidence brought together in this chapter shows that the quality of social relations is better in more equal societies where income differences between rich and poor are smaller. We shall see that in these more equal societies, people are much more likely to trust each other, measures of social capital and social cohesion show that community life is stronger, and homicide rates and levels of violence are consistently lower.

Psychological literature, concentrating as it does on the individual, too often ignores our susceptibility to the powerful sociological processes that drive social differentiation and discrimination against those lower down the social hierarchy. On the other hand, the sociological literature that addresses issues of social class stratification usually ignores its interaction with individual psychology. This book brings individual and society together in an attempt to increase our awareness of some of the most powerful ways in which individual psychology interacts with the wider sociological processes responsible for damaging our humanity and producing dysfunctional societies. Our point of entry into these issues is a recognition that there is a close relationship between inequality and the quality of social relations. Later we shall come to an understanding of the processes responsible for that relationship.

Whether people seem friendly or hostile, whether they are gregarious or keep to themselves, whether they are gentle or violent, trusting or suspicious, whether or not they are involved in local community life—such differences are usually seen as little more than a matter of chance differences in personality arising from some combination of genes and early childhood experience. But we frequently say that people in some places are friendlier, more relaxed, or less violent than people in other places. Usually, the more friendly, relaxed, and safe a place is, the better everyone likes it. In fact, these differences are real enough: the statistics show that there are important differences between societies in how much people trust each other, how likely they are to be involved in community life, and levels of violence. The nature of social relations is a crucial part of the quality of our lives, and there is no doubt that some societies are, quite simply, nicer than others.

If you ask people what makes some places friendlier, the most common suggestion is that it must be a reflection of different cultural traditions. But without knowing what lies behind "cultural traditions" or why they change over time, that is not a very helpful answer; it does not tell us where these different cultural traditions come from or what we can do to make a society friendlier.

In fact, the amount of social and economic inequality between people exerts—as we shall see—a very powerful influence on the quality of social relations. In the modern world it is necessary to prove that the quality of social relations is strongly affected by the amount of inequality, but the link seemed obvious to many people in previous generations. Some of the early Christian socialists advocated greater equality not, as now, simply on the grounds that it is a fairer sharing-out of goods between people whom we have come to see as self-interested consumers, but because they saw it as a crucial step on the road to a greater human harmony and a fuller realization of our inherent sociality. Often calling each other "brother," "sister," or "comrade," they saw differences in wealth and income as the major cause of social divisions in society.

How cohesive a society is, how much people trust each other and are involved in community life, is an important social asset that makes a very substantial contribution to the quality of life. It is usually referred to as "social capital," as if to imply that it is also an economic resource. There is now a great deal of interest from people across the political spectrum in improving the quality of social relations and strengthening involvement in community life. Some of this reflects a concern that there has been a decline in public-spiritedness, in social attitudes and behavior in the public sphere, that has been particularly serious in poorer urban areas. Concerned with government responses to the problems of poverty and deprivation, a few on the political left fear that the concept of social capital is popular because it suggests a cheap way of tackling many of the effects of relative poverty while avoiding facing up to the more expensive task of tackling poverty itself. If—as the data show—social capital is lowest in the most deprived areas (partly as a reflection of higher rates of crime and violence), then politicians may be tempted to believe that it is not more money that people in these poor areas need, but better social relations. Although such a misunderstanding may well explain why social capital is an attractive concept to some on the political right, the truth is exactly the other way around. What the relationship with incquality actually demonstrates is that societies that tolerate the injustices of great inequality will almost inescapably suffer their social consequences: they will be unfriendly and violent societies, recognized more for their hostility than for their hospitality.

While income differences have widened in many countries during the last decades of the twentieth century, there have been signs—at least among a minority of commentators—of a reemergence of the intuitive recognition that inequality is socially corrosive. But despite the widespread—and fashionable—interest in the concept of social capital and the quality of community relations, there has been an almost total failure to recognize the extent to which increases in social capital are dependent on greater equality. This is particularly ironic because the growing interest in social capital is itself the result of a decline in the quality of social relations and in community life reflecting, in large part, the effects of increasing inequality.

The former socialist belief in the benefits of equality is ignored in discussions of practical policy because it appears, at best, as empty idealism, relevant only to those who dream of a utopia in which some perfect human equality has been established and lions lie down with lambs. Few have regarded the benefits of equality as relevant to the small differences in the scale of inequality between existing societies. It comes as a surprise, therefore, to discover that differences in inequality as small as those found between different market democracies or different U.S. states produce very substantial social and health effects.

Tocqueville

One of the earliest works on the strength of community life was Alexis de Tocqueville's *Democracy in America,* in which he describes his visit to America in 1831. Although people writing on social capital often quote his descriptions of the strength of community life in the United States, they always omit what he thought were the reasons for its strength. Even on the first page of his book he makes his views clear:

> Among the new objects that attracted my attention during my stay in the United States, none struck me with greater force than the equality of conditions. I easily perceived the enormous influence that this primary fact exercises on the workings of the society. It gives a particular direction to the public mind, a particular turn to the laws, new maxims to those who govern, and particular habits to the governed.
>
> I soon recognized that this same fact extends its influence far beyond political mores and laws, and that its empire expands over civil society as well as government: it creates opinions, gives rise to sentiments, inspires customs, and modifies everything that it does not produce.
>
> In this way, then, as I studied American society, I saw more and more in the equality of conditions, the generative fact from which each particular fact seemed to flow, and I kept finding that fact before me again and again as a central point to which all of my observations were leading. (2000: 1)

With the French Revolution still in people's recent memory, one of the exciting things about American society for a Frenchman such as Tocqueville was that the United States was a society without a feudal nobility—without the landed aristocracy that Tom Paine had argued in his *Rights of Man* (1792) were the scourge of European society.

Tocqueville also explained the reasons why he thought greater equality led to a stronger civic community life.

> When all men . . . are ranked in an irrevocable way according to their occupation, wealth, and birth, . . . each caste has its opinions, its sentiments, its rights, its moral habits, its separate existence. Thus the men who compose it bear no resemblance to any of the others; they do not have the same way of thinking or of feeling, and if they believe themselves to belong to the same humanity, they do so just barely. . . . When the chroniclers of the Middle Ages, who all, by their birth or their habits, belonged to the aristocracy, report the tragic death of a noble, they express infinite sorrows; whereas they recount in one breath and without batting an eye the massacre and tortures of the common people. (2000: 249)

A couple of pages further on, he adds:

> When ranks are almost equal among a people, with all men having more or less the same manner of thinking and feeling, each of them can judge in an instant the feelings of all the others: he casts a rapid glance at himself; that suffices for him. There is thus no misery that he cannot easily conceive of and whose dimensions are not revealed to him by a secret instinct. It does not matter whether it is a question of strangers or enemies: his imagination puts him immediately in their place. It mixes something personal into his pity and makes him suffer himself when the body of his fellow man is torn apart. (2000: 251)

Rather than ignoring the inequality and brutality of slavery, Tocqueville recognized that slaves "experience horrible miseries and are constantly exposed to extremely cruel punishments," but rather than thinking that weakened his argument, he saw it as proof that inequality played the formative role:

> It is easy to see that the lot of these unfortunates inspires little pity in their masters and that they see in slavery not only a state of affairs from which they profit, but also an evil that scarcely touches them. In this way, the same man who is full of humanity for his fellow men when they are at the same time his equals becomes insensitive to their sufferings the moment the equality ceases. (2000: 251)

Circumstantial Evidence

I first looked to see if there were differences in the quality of social relations in more and less egalitarian societies as part of a search for explanations of why more egalitarian societies were, as we shall see in chapter 4, healthier. I looked for differences between healthier egalitarian societies and less healthy, more unequal ones.

Initially I had little to go on except unquantified circumstantial evidence. But the differences between more and less equal societies were clear enough (Wilkinson 1996a). The evidence suggested that more egalitarian societies were substantially more socially cohesive. I shall mention just three examples here. During the First and Second World Wars, British government policy was designed to foster national unity and a sense that the burden of war was shared equally across the whole society. As Richard Titmuss put it: "If the cooperation of the masses was thought to be essential [to the war effort], then inequalities had to be reduced and the pyramid of social stratification had to be flattened" (Titmuss 1958: 86). Not only did income differences narrow dramatically among those in employment, but unemployment almost disappeared, and income tax became much more progressive. The policy seemed to have had its desired effect: people talked of a strong sense of camaraderie, social cohesion, and common purpose. A remarkable result was that civilian death rates fell two or three times as fast as in other periods during the twentieth century.

Japan and Sweden were the second and third examples I looked at. According to World Bank data, they were (in the 1980s) the most egalitarian countries in the developed world. Japan was also the healthiest country and Sweden the second healthiest in terms of life expectancy. They were both notably cohesive, with low rates of violent crime and high levels of interpersonal trust. Here the contrast with the United States, where trust is low and homicide rates are the highest in the developed world, was inescapable: not only does the United States trail behind most other developed countries in longevity, despite both its wealth and its high expenditure on medical care, but U.S. income differences are the widest of any of the rich developed market democracies.

Trust

Fortunately, data that allow us to go beyond selected examples of this kind have more recently become available. In an attempt to explain why American states with smaller income differences had higher life expectancies, Ichiro Kawachi and Bruce Kennedy (1997) showed that people were much more trusting of each other in more equal states. Using a question from the U.S. General Social Survey, they showed that where income differences were larger, more people believed that others "would take advantage of you if they got the chance." The relation between inequality and this measure of trust is shown in figure 2.1, reproduced from their paper. Between states there are very substantial differences in the proportion of people who say they trust others, and the differences are closely related to inequality. In the most equal states, only 10 or 15 percent of the population feel they cannot trust others, while in the more unequal states the proportion rises to 35 or 40 percent.

Figure 2.1: People do not trust each other where income differences are greater

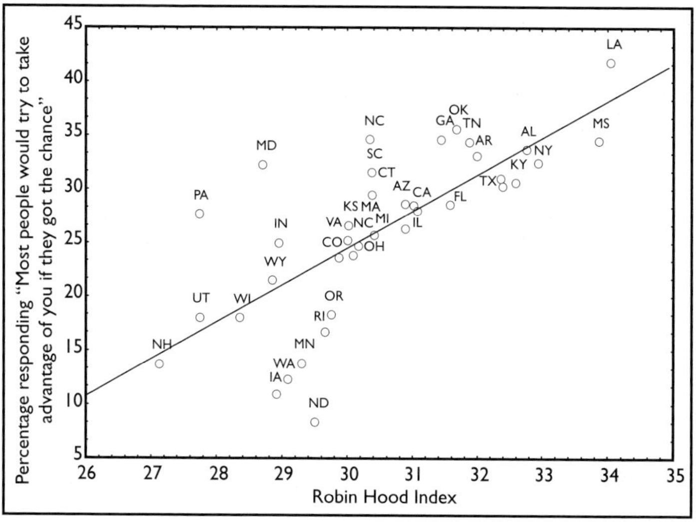

The Robin Hood Index of Income Inequality is the percentage of a society's income that would have to be taken from the rich and given to the poor to get equality. Trust is measured here (on the vertical axis) by the proportion of the population who agree "most people would try to take advantage of you if they got the chance." The graph shows that the proportion of people who do not trust others rises from 10 or 15 percent in the more egalitarian states (on the left) to 35 or 40 percent in the most unequal states (on the right).

Source: I. Kawachi et al., "Social Capital, Income Inequality, and Morality," *American Journal of Public Health* 87 (1997): 1,491–98. Reproduced with permission from the American Public Health Association.

The tendency for a higher proportion of the population in societies with smaller income differences between rich and poor to feel they can trust each other is not just an American phenomenon. In his recent book *The Moral Foundations of Trust,* Eric Uslaner (2002) also drew attention to a tendency for more egalitarian societies to be more trusting. The international relationship he found is shown here in figure 2.2. (Despite appearing to slope in opposite directions in figures 2.1 and 2.2 both relationships show the same pattern: the difference is that the vertical axis in figure 2.1 shows high levels of mistrust at the top, whereas in figure 2.2 high levels of trust are at the top.)

**Figure 2.2: People trust each other less in countries
with larger income differences**

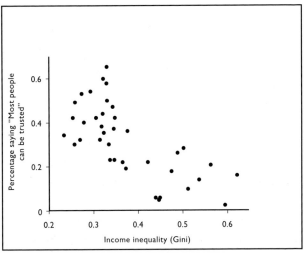

This graph excludes the ex-communist countries. It shows that in countries with more unequal incomes (to the right), a smaller proportion of people agree that "most people can be trusted."

Source: E. Uslaner, *The Moral Foundations of Trust* (New York: Cambridge University Press, 2002). Redrawn with permission of Cambridge University Press.

In addition to these analyses of trust and inequality, Robert Putnam told me (personal communication) that in an unpublished analysis he had found a strong relationship between data on trust taken from the World Values Survey and inequality for a large number of different countries. At one end of the distribution lay Brazil, with among the largest income differences and lowest levels of trust, while at the other was Sweden, with an unusually narrow income distribution and among the highest levels of trust. Rather than being outliers, he emphasized, these two countries were very much part of the relationship shown among other countries.

The Strength of Community Life

It is of course Robert Putnam who more than anyone else has put social capital and people's involvement in community life on the academic and political agenda as an important and measurable component of human welfare. A professor of political science at Harvard, he is recognized as the guru of social capital. His two most important studies (Putnam 2000; Putnam, Leonardi, and Nanetti 1993) are of the United States and of the regions in Italy. In both he measured people's involvement in community life by combining lots of different indicators into a single index of the strength of community life. Most important is the proportion of people belonging to voluntary groups and associations—sports clubs, gardening groups, charitable organizations, Scout troops, choirs, and so on. But also included as indicators of involvement in community life are things such as whether people bother to vote in local elections or read local newspapers.

Putnam's study of social capital in Italy (Putnam, Leonardi, and Nanetti 1993) is an attempt to explain differences in the performance of the twenty regional governments set up in 1970 with the same funding per head of population. Although there was a tendency for governments in the richer regions to do better than others, he found that the quality of local government performance was most closely related to his measures of how involved people are in community life. Despite having little research interest in income inequality, Putnam points out in a footnote (224, n. 52) that his index of "civic community" was very closely related (r = 0.81) to measures of income inequality in each of the twenty Italian regions: participation in community life was much stronger where income differences were smaller.

Putnam also interviewed community leaders and local people in the Italian regions. Talking about social attitudes and an egalitarian social ethos rather than income inequality itself, he says: "Political leaders in the civic regions are more enthusiastic supporters of political equality than their counterparts in less civic regions" (1993: 102). "Citizens in the more civic regions, like their leaders, have a pervasive distaste for hierarchical authority patterns" (104). "Equality is an essential feature of the civic community" (105). He contrasts the "horizontal" social relations in the more civic and egalitarian areas with what he refers to as "vertical," "patron-client" relations in the less civic regions.

Putnam's study of trends in social capital in the United States, called *Bowling Alone,* was published in 2000. In it he shows a clear tendency for the states in the United States that score highest on his index of involvement in community life to be those where income differences are smallest. This cross-sectional relationship, much like the one he found in his Italian study, is shown in figure 2.3.

Figure 2.3: Social capital is higher in
U.S. states in which incomes
are more equal

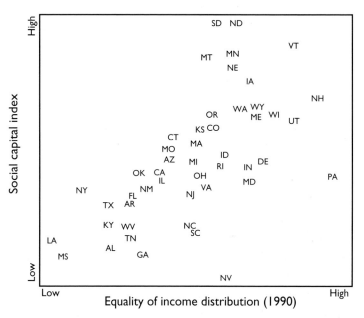

States in which income differences are smaller (on the right here) score higher in Putnam's measure of social capital, showing that people in these states are more in-volved in community life. The most unequal states (to the left) have the lowest levels of involvement in community life.

Source: Transposed from R.D. Putnam, *Bowling Alone: The Collapse and Revival of American Community* (New York: Simon & Schuster, 2000), fig. 92. Reprinted with the permission of Simon & Schuster Adult Publishing Group. Copyright © 2000 by Robert D. Putnam.

However, as well as these pieces of cross-sectional evidence from the United States and Italy, in his American study Putnam looks at changes over time in involvement in community life. Interestingly, although inequality is only peripheral to Putnam's interests, he is keen to allay suspicions that his measures of involvement in community life may only reflect the extent to which people socialize *within* their religious, racial, or class groupings, rather than forming wider links and mixing across them. In order to show that social capital bridges these divides, he points out how trends in social capital and in income differences have almost exactly mirrored each other throughout the last century. He says:

> Community and equality are mutually reinforcing. . . . Social capital and economic inequality moved in tandem through most of the twentieth century. In terms of the distribution of wealth and income, America in the 1950s and 1960s was more egalitarian than it had been in more than a century. . . . [T]hose same decades were also the high point of social connectedness and civic engagement. Record highs in equality and social capital coincided.
>
> Conversely, the last third of the twentieth century was a time of growing inequality and eroding social capital. By the end of the twentieth century the gap between rich and poor in the U.S. had been increasing for nearly three decades, the longest sustained increase in inequality for at least a century. The timing of the two trends is striking: somewhere around 1965–70 America reversed course and started becoming both less just economically and less well connected socially and politically. (2000: 359)

Despite this statement, Putnam has not been especially interested in inequality. He mentions it only as an occasional side issue and has no discussion of why inequality and social capital are related. Nevertheless, a careful reading of his work provides invaluable evidence that the two are linked: first, cross-sectional relationships both among the fifty U.S. states and among the twenty regions of Italy, then a remarkable fit between time trends in equality and involvement in community life in the United States throughout the last century, and finally some survey evidence that civic leaders and populations of regions with higher social capital have more egalitarian or democratic values. In addition to this evidence he has published, Putnam referred in a recent seminar (University College London, March 12, 2003) to other unpublished data analyses he had done, and concluded by saying, "There is absolutely no doubt at all that they [inequality and social capital] are very closely related."

Homicide and Inequality

Perhaps the strongest evidence that the quality of social relations is related to income inequality comes from studies of violent crime and homicide. Legal definitions and published statistics on many different kinds of crime usually differ too much from country to country to allow sound international comparisons. But homicide is an exception: what counts as murder is widely agreed upon, and comparisons between countries are much more straightforward.

There have now been over fifty studies showing a clear tendency for violence to be more common in societies where income differences are larger. The evidence comes from international studies of developed and developing countries as well as from studies of areas within countries, and it stands up to controlling for average income levels as well as for poverty.

Figure 2.4 (taken from Daly et al. 2001) shows the relation among the fifty U.S. states and ten provinces of Canada. It shows at least a tenfold difference in homicide rates related to inequality. The difference is not simply a contrast between the United States and Canada: it holds within each country on its own, and about half of the overall variation in homicide rates seems to be accounted for by differences in the amount of inequality in each state or province.

Figure 2.4: Homicide rates in relation to income inequality among U.S. states and Canadian provinces

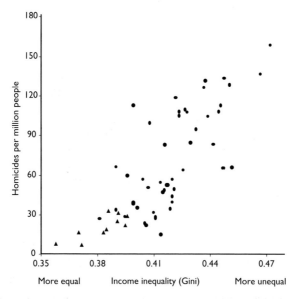

Homicide is more common in more unequal U.S. states (circles) and Canadian provinces (triangles). Bigger income differences are to the right here

Source: M. Daly, M. Wilson, and S. Vasdev, "Income Inequality and Homicide Rates in Canada and the United States," *Canadian Journal of Criminology* 43 (2001): 219–36. Redrawn with permission of the *Canadian Journal of Criminology and Criminal Justice*. Copyright by the Canadian Criminal Justice Association.

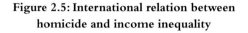

Figure 2.5: International relation between homicide and income inequality

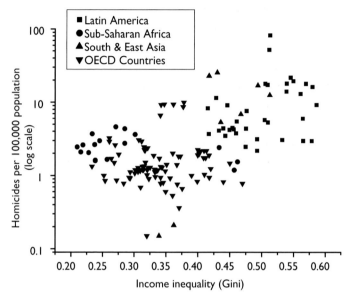

Homicide rates are higher in countries in which income differences are larger (shown to the right). Relationships like this have been demonstrated forty to fifty times.

Source: P. Fajnzylber, D. Lederman, and N. Loayza. "Inequality and Violent Crime." *Journal of Law and Economics* 2002; 45 (1): 1–40. Copyright 2002 by The University of Chicago. All rights reserved.

Fajnzylber and colleagues (2002) found a similar relationship between homicide rates and income inequality, but this time using international data for thirty-nine countries. Figure 2.5 is reproduced from their paper. Although the relationship shown here is still statistically highly significant, part of the reason why it is not as close as that shown in the United States and Canada (figure 2.4) is that the international data—particularly the data on income distribution—is much less accurate and much less comparable.

Even as long ago as 1993 there were over forty published studies of this relationship, of which some thirty-four provided the necessary data to be included in a metanalysis. Writing in the *Criminal Justice Review*, the authors of that study (Hsieh and Pugh 1993) concluded that the relationship between inequality and violence was a robust one. They also said poverty was independently associated with higher levels of violence. While this may well be true, particularly in the poorer countries, some of the evidence on which that conclusion was based looked at low income in small areas in a way that did not show whether the association was really with absolute levels of poverty or with poverty relative to the wider society. If we were, for instance, to ask why areas such as Harlem in New York had such high levels of violence, the answer is less likely to be that the absolute level of poverty in Harlem is the true cause rather than the fact that people in Harlem are poor *in relation* to people in the rest of the United States.

So firmly established is the relationship between inequality and homicide—at least in the research literature if not in the minds of politicians and the public—that many criminologists regard it as the most well-established relation between homicide and *any* environmental factor. Among recent comments in the academic literature to that effect are the following:

> [T]he most consistent finding in cross-national research on homicides has been that of a positive association between income inequality and homicides. (Neapolitan 1999: 260)

> A finding that has emerged with remarkable consistency is that high rates of homicide tend to accompany high levels of

inequality in the distribution of income. (Messner and Rosenfeld 1997: 1,394)

[E]conomic inequality is positively and significantly related to rates of homicide despite an extensive list of conceptually relevant controls. The fact that this relationship is found with the most recent data and using a different measure of economic inequality from previous research, suggests that the finding is very robust. (Lee and Bankston 1999: 50)

Hostility, Racism, and Voting

Closely fitting the evidence on violence are the results of an analysis of average hostility levels in ten U.S. cities (Williams, Feaganes, and Barefoot 1995; Williams, personal communication). The Cook-Medley Hostility Scale in the Minnesota Multiphasic Personality Inventory was administered to random samples of two hundred people in each city, and an average hostility score was calculated for each city. Using these data, which Williams kindly let me see, I found the relationship ($r = 0.68$, $p < 0.05$) between average hostility measures and income inequality in these ten cities shown in figure 2.6.

In a paper entitled "Disrespect and Black Mortality" Kennedy and Kawachi found that measures of racial prejudice in the fifty U.S. states were also strongly related to income inequality (Kennedy and Kawachi 1997). Several studies show that women's status also suffers—both in terms of political participation and in terms of their earnings disadvantage relative to men—in societies where there is a larger gap between rich and poor (Blau and Kahn 1992; Kawachi et al. 1999). What greater income inequality, more discrimination against

Figure 2.6: Hostility levels are lower in more equal cities

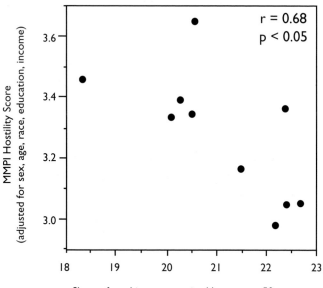

Share of total income received by poorest 50 percent

Average hostility levels in ten U.S. cities (assessed in a random sample of people in each) are lower in the cities (lower right in figure) where a higher proportion of income goes to the poorest half of the population.

Source: R.B. Williams, J. Feaganes, and J.C. Barefoot, "Hostility and Death Rates in 10 U.S. Cities." *Psychosomatic Medicine* 1995; 57 (1): 94, and personal communication.

women, and discrimination against ethnic minorities all have in common is that they all involve a greater exploitation of power differentials to the disadvantage of lower status and weaker groups, whether defined by ethnicity, gender, or social class. (We shall discuss this further in chapter 7.)

Lastly, there is a growing literature showing that a smaller proportion of people bother to vote in elections in more unequal societies. This seems to be true not only at the national level, but also in analyses of inequality and voting within subnational regions (Mahler 2002; Blakely, Kennedy, and Kawachi 2001). As well as being seen as related to the tendency for involvement in community life to be lower where there is more inequality, this is probably part of a wider tendency for mistrust of government to increase as the gap between "them" and "us" widens with greater inequality.

Summing Up

All these studies together provide very substantial evidence that, at least in modern societies, the quality of social relations is poorer where income differences are bigger. As well as examples such as Britain during the two world wars, Sweden, Japan, and the United States, we also have statistical evidence about trust (internationally as well as within the United States); on involvement in community life cross-sectionally in the United States and in Italy and over time in the United States; on hostility in U.S. cities; on homicide both within countries as well as internationally; and on discrimination against women and ethnic minorities. Although a disproportionate amount of this evidence comes from the United States (no doubt partly because the United States is one of the few countries to collect reliable income data as part of its census, enabling researchers to calculate income distribution figures for areas within the United States), there is still plenty—particularly from studies of homicide, violent crime, and trust—to show that these relationships are far from confined to the United States.

Only one research paper appears to detract partially from this picture. Lynch and colleagues (2001) reported that there was no relationship between inequality and associational life among a group of developed countries. However, their results reflected only their failure to separate out the transitional economies of Eastern Europe. As these countries were then undergoing a traumatic social and economic breakdown following the collapse of communism and had no tradition of independent civic associations, no voluntary sector or strength of community life, it was hardly surprising that they had low levels of social capital compared to the well-ordered societies of Western Europe.

Although trust, involvement in community life, homicide, and hostility differ widely, we cannot plausibly regard these measures as completely independent of each other. It is much more likely that they are all different measures of underlying variations in the quality of social relationships. The fact that they are all related to inequality indicates a general shift in the tenor of social relations associated with larger or smaller differences in income. Places with high homicide rates would then be places where we would also expect to find more hostility, lower levels of trust, and less involvement in community life. This means that instead of regarding homicide as a bizarre form of behavior, unrelated to others, we should see it as the extreme end of a continuum of relationships which run all the way from the most kindly, supportive, and trusting to the most hostile and violent. The implication is perhaps that the whole balance, or center of gravity, of relationships is different in different societies, so that the quality of social relations right across a society is shifted either toward the gentler, more affiliative end of the spectrum or toward the more antisocial and violent end.

Health research provides a model of how we should perhaps think of the character of different kinds of relationships in a society as shifting together, so that people in some societies treat each other a little better—whether at home, at work, or in the street—and in others a little worse. Geoffrey Rose (1992) found such a model fitted the distribution of a range of health risk factors in some thirty-two different societies. He looked, for example, at the proportion who were heavy drinkers, were obese, had high blood pressure, or suffered serious cognitive impairment in later life. For each of these he found that the proportion of such people was a function, respectively, of the society's average alcohol consumption, average ratio of weight to height, average blood pressure, and so on. Rather than finding that most people in all societies drank similar amounts and that what varied was simply the proportion who drank much more than the average, he found almost the opposite: that societies with a lot of alcoholics were always societies where most people drank more, and the average alcohol consumption very accurately predicted the number of alcoholics. In a similar way, societies in which there were more people with dangerously high blood pressure did not just have more people at the extreme, but most people's blood pressure was higher. With each of these health risk factors the proportions at dangerously high levels were not odd minorities behaving differently from the rest of the society but were part of a behavioral shift to which the norms of the whole of the rest of society seemed to contribute.

It looks as if the same picture is likely to be true for different measures of the quality of social relationships. Because more unequal places are marked by a more conflictual character of social relationships—so that they suffer not only more homicide, but also more violent crime, less trust, less involvement in community life, and more racism—we should see them all as part of a single continuum affecting the nature of social relations throughout a society. Inequality seems to shift the whole distribution of social relationships away from the most affectionate end toward the more conflictual end, so that, given what we know from the available data, we might also expect people in more unequal societies would turn out to be less helpful to strangers and less considerate to junior employees, and that there would be more conflict in school playgrounds and perhaps more domestic conflict and more prejudice against disadvantaged groups.

We shall leave the discussion of *why* the quality of social relations is related to the extent of income inequality, and which way causality goes, until chapters 5 and 6.

What is at stake here is hugely important to the quality of life in modern societies. The tone of social relations is one of the most fundamental determinants of the real quality of life, and if, as the evidence seems to suggest, social relations are strongly affected by the extent of income inequality, this holds out the exciting possibility that there are clear instruments of public policy that could be used to produce major population-wide improvements in social life and psychosocial well-being.

To explain what is going on in these relationships we need to understand more about how we interact with our social environment and what aspects of it we find stressful. As we saw in the first chapter, health research provides an important source of insights because psychosocial risk factors, working through stress, have such a powerful impact on health. The next chapter outlines the main psychosocial risk factors for poor health, after which chapter 4 goes on to show how health too is harmed by greater income inequality.

3
Anxieties and Insecurities
The Eyes of Others

This chapter lays the foundations for understanding how we, as individuals, can be affected by inequality in ways that lead more unequal societies to have the higher levels of violence and reduced levels of trust and involvement in community life we saw in the last chapter. Although we won't build on these foundations until chapters 5 and 6, they need to be established here in order to prepare for chapter 4, which shows how average standards of health are higher in more egalitarian societies. The problem is to understand what it is about us, as human beings, which means that inequality can affect both health and the quality of social relations. Here we shall see not only the basic nature of our sensitivity to the social world but how, through that, it comes to affect us biologically.

In chapter 1 we described the scale of "health inequalities" found within countries throughout the developed world. We pointed out that, depending on the extent of socioeconomic inequalities in a society, the average life expectancy among poorer and less well-educated people might be anything from two to fifteen years shorter than among people nearer the top of the social pyramid. We also saw that rather than being a simple health difference between the poor and the rest of society, the normal pattern is that longevity increases all the way up the social hierarchy to the top.

Instead of attracting urgent government attention in every country, remarkably few governments have pursued policies intended to reduce the tens of thousands of extra deaths lower down the social hierarchy that contribute to health inequalities. The Whitehall Study of civil servants working in London offices, which showed that death rates were, age for age, three times as high among the most junior office workers compared to the most senior, has not led to urgent attempts to remove the causes of the excess deaths. If people were dying from exposure to some toxic material, the offices would be instantly closed down until the danger had been removed. But because these deaths are caused by social processes, there is none of the same sense of urgency. Social toxicity attracts less attention than exposure to less dangerous chemical hazards, and it is easier to vacate contaminated buildings than to change social structures. We could speculate on how different the response would be if the slope of the social gradient in death and disease ran in the opposite direction, so the highest-status people did the worst. That would at least be fairer—the shortening of life could then be seen as the price the privileged pay for the higher quality of life they enjoy, rather than as an additional burden associated with a poorer quality of life. If health inequalities were the other way around, we might expect analyses of whether the economy could withstand the cost of losing an average of five or ten years of life expectancy among its brightest and best captains of industry.

The health differences are not primarily a reflection of differences in medical care. In Britain, where medical care is free, poorer people tend to use medical services more than richer people. The question is whether they use them enough to offset their greater burden of disease, not whether their greater burden of disease comes from worse access to medical care. In fact, the effects of any differences in medical care are dwarfed by differences in who gets heart disease and cancer and who is injured on the roads. Although there are class differences in survival rates once you have any of these conditions (Leon and Wilkinson 1989), their impact is smaller than the impact of the differences in who gets what to start with. To understand the position of medical care in relation to the overall burden of disease in a population, you need to think of it as functioning rather like an army medical corps. Though it is essential to have good medical treatment for battle casualties, if you want to know why the number of casualties in a war was large or small, you need to look at the nature of the battle, not at the medical corps. In society at large, the nature of the battle, which would explain overall health standards, is the nature of social and economic life. It is not that medical care is ineffective, but rather that its effectiveness is a minor influence compared to the socioeconomic factors which establish the initial burden of disease. The Office of Health Economics (1992, 1993) used to publish a graph showing the number of prescription items per head of population in relation to levels of unemployment for administrative areas of England and Wales. There was a very strong tendency (r = 0.8) for areas with higher unemployment to receive many more medical prescriptions; in effect, rather than the medical care system determining levels of health, the nature of social and economic life determines the burden of disease which the medical system then has to cope with.

When I first became interested in the social gradient in health some twenty-five years ago, I, like most researchers working on this problem, assumed that the health differences we saw between different occupational classes resulted from differences in material living standards. (As mentioned in chapter 1, studies had shown that differences in health-related behavior—differences in drinking, smoking, exercise, and so on—failed to account for the bulk of the health differences.) Most of us assumed our task was to identify what aspects of the differences in material living standards contributed to which diseases. But what has become clear from numerous studies over the years is the surprising success of *psychosocial* variables in explaining differences in morbidity and mortality. Variables such as a lack of a sense of control, depression, hopelessness, hostility, lack of confidence, lack of social support, bad social relationships, stressful life events, family conflict, stress at work, social and material rewards from work that fail to match work effort, bereavement, being single or divorced rather than married, and job and housing insecurity all seemed to produce poor health.

Many psychological variables are regarded as a matter of chance differences in individual character traits and circumstances. We rarely think about how they might be affected by social structure and social position. But people's psychological states are highly situational and therefore socially structured. Although each person has his or her unique psychology, we are all affected by circumstances, by common patterns of meaning in our society, and by the impact of social structures on our emotional and psychological life. The term *psychosocial* is often used in preference to *psychological* to emphasize the extent to which the features of emotional life that affect health are socially patterned and dependent on the social context rather than simply on individual happenstance.

The shift in emphasis from individual psychology to the social patterning of psychological life reflects the fact that epidemiological studies of health and health inequalities often collect data from many thousands, sometimes tens of thousands, of people. The interest is inevitably in the broad patterns rather than the individual differences. But at the same time the broad patterns tell us more about individual sensitivities. When we see, for instance, that levels of stress hormones in middle age are related to birth weight, or—as in the last chapter—that levels of violence and the quality of social relationships in a society are related to the degree of inequality, we are learning about processes which affect individuals. Often they are processes we may be blind to until we see the evidence in data comparing large numbers of people.

Some of these relationships are obvious enough. If you don't have enough money, if your job is at risk, or if you can't pay off your debts, then you feel anxious and worry about it. In examples of this kind, the sources of stress are clear enough; even to talk about the "social patterning" of psychosocial risk seems to be making a mystery where there is none. But even in cases such as these there can be confusion as to whether the processes are material or psychosocial. Job insecurity seems an external material factor, yet it affects health through the worry it causes. The same is true of debt. The normal basis on which we distinguish between material and psychosocial factors hinges on whether the health impact is dependent on some conscious or unconscious perception or cognitive processing, or whether, in contrast, it affects health regardless of what we think or feel or know. So, for instance, things such as air pollution, infectious microorganisms, poisoning, and vitamin deficiencies are all capable of harming our health even if we are totally unaware of them: they are therefore classified as material factors having a direct effect on health. But job or housing insecurity affects your health only if you are aware of it. Similarly, the practical causes of feelings of hostility, depression, or lack of a sense of control may be clear enough, but if it is those *feelings* that are doing the health damage, they are classified as psychosocial, even if the remedies are often material. That is an important point: the remedies for psychosocial stressors often involve changes in material circumstances. Because they are classified according to the pathways through which health effects are transmitted, psychosocial factors would allow us to ignore material circumstances only in a world where people's thoughts, feelings, worries, and anxieties were entirely independent of practical life. But we do not live in such an absurd world: psychosocial factors reflect material life because material life is a source of stress, whether in the form of unhappiness, depression, insecurity, anger, or anxiety.

Despite individual differences, mental states are rarely independent of the practical world. Instead they are perceptions of it and attempts to make sense of one's situation in it. Sometimes an emphasis on psychosocial influences on health is criticized for seeming unrelated to the practical reality of people's lives: what is at stake is, however, their experience of life, and the easiest way to change that is to change the practical reality. But to know what to change we need to know the way people's worlds are subjectively constructed and experienced, and that is why the psychosocial is crucial. The growing understanding of the biological pathways through which stress affects health has provided us with one more major new pathway through which the environment can affect health. It is no longer just a matter of what we ingest or inhale, or how we use our bodies; it is also a matter of our feelings and subjective experience of life.

Much of the research trying to understand socioeconomic influences on health started out from the social patterning of health underlying health inequalities. Health inequalities provided compelling evidence of the extraordinary sensitivity of health to socioeconomic factors. Our task had two components: first, to identify more accurately what it was about social status differences that affected health so powerfully, and second, to understand how those factors influence our biology and vulnerability to disease. This latter component is discussed in chapter 8 and largely concerns the biological effects of chronic stress. In the current chapter we will address the first part of the problem. We will discuss what have emerged as the three most important categories of psychosocial risk to have been identified: the effects of high or low social status, being more socially isolated rather than embedded in strong friendship networks, and the influence of early emotional and social development.

Concentrating on these psychosocial influences does not mean that the direct effects of poorer material circumstances do not matter. Things such as poor diet, air pollution, smoking, and bad housing obviously do matter. But we should not be too simplistic about them and imagine that there are very clear connections between, for instance, exposure to the physical hazards of poor-quality housing and the causation of cancers or heart disease. Similarly, economic factors such as low income or unemployment, which might be seen as having a direct material influence on health, may well have their main health effects through the psychosocial stress of feeling stigmatized and looked down on or feeling angry and ashamed at being devalued.

Lastly, although health-related behavior, including smoking, drinking, and not exercising, clearly does have a direct impact on health, there are undoubtedly powerful psychosocial factors explaining why poorer people smoke more and take less leisure-time exercise. No one can be unaware of the times when each of us needs more of the props with which we try to comfort and console ourselves, the times when we drink more, start "eating for comfort," or are most likely to start smoking again. Keeping to the dos and don'ts of healthy behavior often means making resolutions that feel like self-denial, and our chances of mustering the necessary willpower are strongly affected by whether we feel on top of our lives or are feeling ground down and in need of substitutes for the comfort, relaxation, and support we lack.

As we are about to see, the psychosocial difficulties leading to poor health spring predominantly from the social environment. Indeed, they show that the social environment is the primary source of stress in modern societies, and the research reveals (with a bit of reading between the lines) how the problems are generated. The important effects of not having adequate power and resources to control one's circumstances, being made to feel inferior, depression, hostility, and lack of support from a friendly social network are central not only to the emerging picture of the determinants of health, but also to understanding why the quality of social life in modern societies has not kept pace with improvements in material life. The psychosocial determinants of health point to the sources of difficulty in our social experience and relationships and provide a unique opportunity to understand not just individual unhappiness but the wider human costs of the social structure.

The fact that this group of extraordinarily powerful psychosocial factors has come to our attention *because* of their impact on health is perhaps little more than a historical accident. The stresses of life to which they draw our attention are important not only because stress causes ill health. They are important primarily because things such as anxiety, depression, lack of support, and feeling looked down on represent subjective suffering. Psychosocial influences on health are not like the health risks of eating too much fatty food—enjoyable but better avoided because of the health effects. Psychosocial factors are important because they go to the heart of our subjective experience of the quality of life. They matter not just because of their health consequences, but in themselves. If you are depressed, you want your depression to end because it is an unhappy state to be in, not merely because someone tells you that it is also a risk factor for heart disease.

One other point about the particular importance of psychosocial risk factors is that the pathways involving chronic stress through which they operate do not just affect health. As we shall see, closely related pathways rooted in relative deprivation also affect a wide range of other problems, including how affiliative or violent people are, the amount of racial and class prejudice, the frequency of dependency on alcohol and other drugs, teenage pregnancies, the educational performance of schoolchildren, behavioral problems in childhood . . . the list goes on.

In contrast, gaining an understanding of the direct *material* causes of ill health would not take us to the heart of the social malaise of modern society and so does not have the same potential to improve the psychosocial well-being of whole populations. The more important direct effects of material factors are already better understood, despite being less powerful, and many of them could be dealt with—provided there is the political will—simply by ensuring that the benefits of economic growth extended to all sections of society.

We will now look in turn at each of the three most powerful categories of psychosocial influences on population health: low social status, weak social affiliations, and emotional difficulties early in life.

Social Status

First social status and position in the social hierarchy. Social position has overwhelmingly powerful consequences. As Simon Charlesworth (2000) says:

> Living in a working class area it is impossible not to confront the presence of a powerful force touching all of our lives; whether it be a force that drives one to steal, be violent, use drugs, suffer mental illness or be quiet, resigned to misery, or, the most usual response, going out to forget one's problems (with drink or drugs), there is something at work in our society that has affected the working class very deeply, that has created fear, insecurity and disillusionment. (196)

While this is a description of what low social status means in a town in the industrial Midlands of Britain, it is just as true of the poorer parts of many cities in the United States and other countries.

Researchers have been slow to recognize the power of the same force to affect health. We struggled to find material factors that could explain why death rates could be anything from two to four times higher in poorer areas than richer ones, and were slow to accept the importance of psychosocial risk factors influenced by the social environment. Despite a growing body of epidemiological literature showing the impact of psychosocial factors on health, we still failed to see that social status is about so much more than better or worse material conditions. And even now few recognize the truth of the remark made by the anthropologist Marshall Sahlins: "Poverty is not a certain small amount of goods, nor is it just a relation between means and ends; above all it is a relation between people. Poverty is a social status. . . . It has grown with civilization . . . as an invidious distinction between classes" (Sahlins 1974: 37).

If the lower levels of health in poorer areas resulted predominantly from the direct effects of lower material living standards, then we would expect to find a clear international relationship between health and living standards from one country to another. In the poorer developing nations we do. Where living standards are too low to provide such basics as clean water and adequate nutrition, then raising living standards improves health. But as countries get richer and fewer people go without basic necessities, the relationship between measures of average living standards—such as gross domestic product per capita (GDPpc)—and health progressively weakens. As figure 3.1 shows, the relation between average income, or GDPpc (on the horizontal axis), and life expectancy (on the vertical axis) is strongest in the poorest countries. As societies get richer during the process of economic development, the

Figure 3.1: Life expectancy in relation
to living standards in rich and poor countries

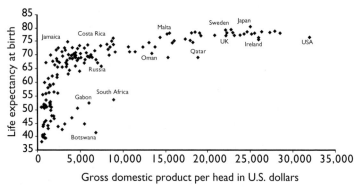

To reflect living standards more accurately, gross domestic product has been converted into 1999 U.S. dollars, taking account of prices in each country. The graph shows that rises in living standards make large differences to life expectancy in poor countries, but make very little difference in rich countries.

curve flattens out and further increases in living standards gradually lose their power to improve standards of health. Among the richest countries, we find no relation whatsoever between GDPpc and average life expectancy: life expectancy in countries as rich as the United States is lower than in most of the other developed countries—worse even than in countries such as Greece that (even after allowing for price differences) are only half as rich. Using data from the World Health Organization for 1998 shows that, among the richest twenty-five countries in the world, not only is there no significant relation between being richer and having better health standards, but the tendency is actually slightly the other way around ($r = -0.107$). For the thirty richest countries, there is still no sign whatsoever of a correlation, significant or not. Only when poorer countries are added in is it possible to find a positive relation, but that is not a sound basis on which to judge the factors affecting health in a country as rich as the United States.

However, despite the lack of any connection between differences in average living standards and health *between* the developed countries, when we look *within* any of them, we find overwhelming evidence of the familiar social gradient in health: people nearer the bottom of the social hierarchy have consistently worse health than those nearer the top. Although the average health of the populations of the rich developed countries does not seem to be affected by large national differences in living standards, within each country health seems finely graded by income. What are we to make of this paradox—a close relationship between income and health *within* each of the richest countries, but not *between* them? Much the most plausible interpretation, and one that fits a much wider body of evidence, is that what matters within countries is not absolute income but income relative to others—a marker of social status and position in society.

If, instead of looking at the international data, we look just at the fifty U.S. states, we find exactly the same picture. Figure 3.2 shows that although there are large differences in average incomes between states—some are nearly twice as rich as others—those differences are unrelated to death rates. Indeed, if you control for the amount of income inequality in each state, the suggestion of the weak, nonsignificant correlation visible in the graph disappears completely. As we shall see in the next chapter, there is a strong relationship between death rates and income inequality in each state.

Important to understanding the connection between in-

Figure 3.2: Death rates (male and female combined) in relation to median income among fifty U.S. states

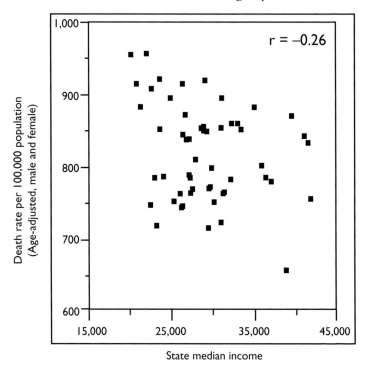

State median income

Although this graph shows a tendency for states with higher incomes per head to have lower death rates, this relation is not statistically significant and disappears completely after controlling for income distribution.

Source: R.G. Wilkinson, "Health Inequalities: Relative or Absolute Standards?" *British Medical Journal* 314 (1997): 591–95. With permission from the BMJ Publishing Group.

come and health within societies is knowing what living standards we are talking about. How do the less well-off in richer societies live? If one looks at government surveys showing ownership of durable consumer goods in different income groups, it is remarkable what a high proportion—even of the poorest 20 percent of the population—own various items. Take Britain, for example. It is not as rich or as unequal as the United States, though it is one of the most unequal societies in Western Europe. Yet if we look at ownership of durable consumer goods among the poorest 20 percent of households in Britain (see table 3.1), we find that 80 percent of the poor own each of the following goods: color television, freezer or refrigerator-freezer, washing machine, central heating, telephone, VCR, and microwave. Even among the newer kinds of goods, over 70 percent have a cell phone. The reason why having an older car, a smaller freezer, or a less smart cell phone is related to health is not because they have direct effects on health; it is because of the social stigma attached to lower material standards. Second-rate goods seem to tell people you are a second-rate person. To believe otherwise is to fundamentally misunderstand the pain of relative poverty or low social status.

Nor should we forget that the problem of health inequalities is not a problem of the poor or the bottom 20 percent compared to the rest of the population, but a gradient in health standards that goes all the way up the social scale.

A second powerful piece of evidence pointing to the importance of social status comes from research on the physiological effects of social status differences among monkeys. Among humans it is almost impossible to make a sharp distinction between differences in material standards based on income and wealth and differences in status, power, and prestige. Those with high status are almost always rich, while those at the bottom of the status hierarchy are almost always poor—so much so that wealth and poverty are an important part of how we assess status. Even occupations such as the

Table 3.1

Percentage of the poorest and richest 20 percent of the population with access to various durable consumer goods, Britain 2002

	Ownership among poorest 20 percent	Ownership among richest 20 percent
Color television	98	99
Freezer/refrigerator-freezer	94	97
Washing machine	93	98
Central heating	89	97
Telephone	87	98
VCR	87	96
Microwave	83	90
CD player	71	95
Cell phone	67	93
Car or van	59	94
Tumble dryer	50	68
Home computer	40	80
Digital television	26	37
Dishwasher	17	59
Satellite dish	13	16
Cable television	11	12

Source: Department for Work and Pensions, *Households Below Average Income 2001/2*, Office for National Statistics (London, 2003).

clergy or priesthood, in which incomes have slipped dramatically relative to the rest of the population over the last century, have been unable to avoid a parallel decline in their social status.

Although it is hard to distinguish between the effects of status and material standards among humans, under experimental conditions it is possible to make an unambiguous distinction between them among species of monkeys that form dominance hierarchies. Experiments have been done which ensured that material conditions are the same for all members of a troop, regardless of whether they were dominant or subordinate. Among others, Carol Shively has studied the physiological effects of social status among captive macaques (Shively and Clarkson 1994). To ensure that material conditions were the same, monkeys of different status lived in the same compounds and were fed the same diet. Social status was experimentally manipulated by moving animals between troops. High-status animals in each group were taken out and put in compounds together so that some had to lose status and become subordinate. Similarly, low-status animals were taken out of their groups and put together so that some would have to become dominant. Shively then measured the resulting physiological changes.

Although we should be reluctant to infer too much from patterns among animals for the human world, what is important about this work is that Shively found a number of physiological effects of low social status among monkeys that are also found to be associated with low social status among humans. These included a much more rapid buildup of arteriosclerosis, a worse ratio of high- to low-density blood fats, and a tendency toward both central obesity and insulin resistance (a precursor to diabetes). The animals that moved down the social scale suffered a fivefold increase in atherosclerosis during the twenty-one months spent in their new social group. Moreover, because the experimental conditions meant there were no material differences between ranks that could explain the results, the findings can only be attributed to low social status itself.

Among the monkeys there can be little doubt that the physiological effects of low social rank were attributable to the stressfulness of subordinate status itself. The subordinate animals are nervous little animals, always having to keep out of the way of and avoid offending their bigger and stronger superiors. To avoid being attacked, subordinates must be submissive and conciliatory, yet despite their best efforts they nevertheless end up with many more bite marks than more dominant animals. Studying baboons in the wild, Robert Sapolsky took measurements of basal levels of cortisol—one of the central stress hormones—and found that lower-ranking animals had higher levels than higher-ranking animals (Sapolsky 1993), confirming that they were more highly stressed. The low-ranking animals also had less healthy (lower) ratios of high- to low-density lipoproteins, adding to the risk of heart disease. Prolonged stress has also been shown to lead to poorer immune function. Margareta Kristenson (Kristenson et al. 1998) found clear social gradients in cortisol levels among men in both Linkoping, Sweden, and Vilnius, Lithuania. She was trying to explain why coronary heart disease was four times as common in Vilnius as in Linkoping. After finding that other risk factors were surprisingly similar, she concluded that the differences in cortisol responses she discovered were an important part of the explanation, not only for the health differences between the two cities, but also for the social class differences in health within each city.

We might feel it would be a mistake to take the comparisons between these findings in animals and people too seriously. But when many of the same physiological differences found to be related to social status among humans are found to be caused by those status differences among nonhuman primates, especially when the experimental conditions rule out explanations in terms of differences in diet and material conditions, it would be foolish to ignore them. And although animal ranking systems and human social stratification seem so different, at bottom they are, as the psychologist Paul Gilbert (1992) points out, both social dominance systems that are about using power to gain preferential access to scarce resources—which is of course why the powerful are rich.

When discussing the distinction between material and psychosocial risk factors earlier in this chapter, I mentioned things such as worries about money, housing, and job insecurity. But this was not why the low-status monkeys were stressed. For monkeys and humans low social status is a stressor in itself: as we shall see (particularly in chapters 5 and 6), we are highly sensitive to feeling looked down on, being devalued, and being treated as second-rate.

Part of this picture are the studies showing that an important health risk factor and contributor to health inequalities is not having the freedom to decide how you do your work. After controlling for numerous other factors, people with less control over their work have much higher death rates (Bosma et al. 1998; Hemingway, Kuper, and Marmot 2002). If you do not exercise control over your work yourself, it is probably because someone else is telling you what to do. Even if something mechanical, like the speed of a production line, prevented you from exercising control over your work, you would probably be blaming someone for running it too fast. Sense of control is a more social concept than is often realized, and it is often affected by how much you are subordinated to the authority and instructions of superiors. We do not experience natural limitations on what we can do—such as our inability to fly or to walk through brick walls—as limitations on our sense of control. But if someone uses his or her power and authority to forbid or prevent us from doing something, then we experience that as a loss of control. At bottom it is about social relations. A strong sense of control comes close to a sense of autonomy. The effects of whether or not people have control over their work should probably be seen as the fine grain of the relation between social status and health, showing our sensitivity to the extent to which we experience our subordination to superiors. This interpretation is supported by research findings showing that a weaker sense of control at work is associated with negative relationships with coworkers and supervisors, and higher levels of anger and hostility (Williams et al. 1997).

It is because the health effects of poverty in developed countries are not primarily the direct results of the physical hazards of lower living standards that there can be dramatic mismatches between living standards and health when we compare groups of people in different societies. In 1996 black American males had a median income of $26,522 and a life expectancy of only 66.1 years. Males in Costa Rica had a mean income (adjusted for price differences) of only $6,410, yet their life expectancy was 75 years. Four times as much real income in the United States bought nine years *less* life expectancy. The explanation for the poorer health of U.S. blacks must have more to do with the psychosocial effects of relative deprivation—educational disadvantage, racism, and other social effects of life in the poorer parts of U.S. cities—than with the direct effects of material standards themselves.

Another example that makes the same point is the health of the Hispanic population of the United States. Although Hispanics are so predominantly poor and, because they come from poorer countries, often have less education than African

Americans, they nevertheless have health that compares well with non-Hispanic whites in the United States. The fact that the Hispanic population of the United States runs counter to such a well-established trend as the tendency for lower-status groups to have poorer health is known as the "Hispanic paradox." Such groups are rare, but their existence shows that there is no automatic relationship between poorer health and either poorer material living standards or poorer education. Where they exist, the key seems to be that they are insulated from suffering a strong sense of their inferior social status by speaking a separate language from their host community. Instead of experiencing themselves simply as poor Americans, Hispanics seem to exist partly as a society within a society, knit together by a separate shared language. Another, much smaller-scale American example, well known to health researchers, was the Italian community in Pennsylvania called Roseto (Bruhn and Wolf 1979). While the Rosetans continued to speak Italian, their health was much better than neighboring towns, despite diets and health-related behaviors that were not advantageous. However, as a generation of Rosetans grew up speaking English and fully integrated into American society, they began to lose their health advantage (Egolf et al. 1992).

While pointing out that the association between poverty and poor health reflects the fact that the poor suffer low social status, it is important to note that researchers studying Roseto ascribed its earlier health advantage to its strong egalitarian sense of community. "[I]t was difficult to distinguish, on the basis of dress and behavior, the wealthy from the impecunious in Roseto. Living arrangements—houses and cars—were simple and strikingly similar. . . . [T]here was no atmosphere of 'keeping up with the Joneses.' . . . [T]he camaraderie among the Italians precluded ostentation or embarrassment to the less affluent" (Buhn and Wolf 1979). The community seemed to lack the material inequalities and social status divisions that make people feel poor.

If the association between health and poverty emanates from the direct biological effects of exposure to poorer material conditions, then it would be hard to explain why exposure to poorer conditions would sometimes fail to affect health. If the main burden of ill health came from breathing polluted air, eating a poor diet, and living in substandard housing, then the health effects of living in those conditions would be almost inescapable. If, however, the health effects are the effects of low social status, then we can see how their impact could occasionally be offset by a sense of community, by a sense of identity, by differences in the frame of reference for social comparisons, by whether you saw yourself as a poor American or a rich Mexican, or by a multitude of other changes in the social meaning of one's circumstances. But in practice the relationship between low social status and poorer material standards is all too robust, and naturally occurring exceptions such as the ones given above are the rare instances that prove the rule.

Friendship

The second of the three main groups of psychosocial risk factors for poor health concerns friendship. An impressive variety of different pieces of research have found that according to almost any measure of social connectedness—such as numbers of friends, whether we have any close confiding relationships, or whether we are involved in community life—social involvement seems strongly beneficial to health.

The earliest work showing the importance of friendship to health comes from the late 1970s (Berkman and Syme 1979; Cassel 1976). In 1988 Jim House and others reviewed five studies of this relationship and found that death rates among both men and women were higher among those who were less socially integrated. As figure 3.3 shows, the results varied from study to study, but overall they average out to suggest that a doubling of risk among more socially isolated people is not an unrepresentative finding.

Typically, studies of the importance of social relationships have controlled for factors like income and education which might confuse the picture. To make quite sure that they were recording the effect of social contact on health rather than the obvious tendency for prior sickness to curtail social life, studies have also excluded from the analysis people who had poor health at the beginning of the study. What they show is that, in a sample of healthy people, those who initially had good social relations are less likely to get ill and die.

The evidence on the importance of friendship does not come from observational studies of the general population alone. Several studies show that survival rates after having had a heart attack may be three times as high among people with good social support (Berkman 1995). Perhaps the most remarkable evidence of the relation between friendship and health comes from a series of experiments conducted by Sheldon Cohen and colleagues (1997). Cohen administered nasal drops containing five different strains of virus for the common cold to a group of 276 healthy volunteers between eighteen and fifty-five years of age. He also collected data on

Figure 3.3: Social connectedness benefits health

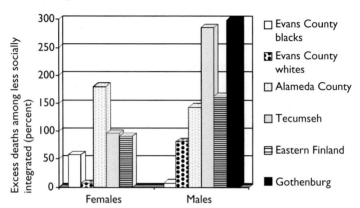

Using data from five community studies, this graph shows how much good social relationships benefit health. It shows the percentage by which death rates among more isolated people exceeded death rates among people with strong social connections in each study. Although sometimes the benefits were small, death rates were often 100 or 200 percent higher among more isolated people.

Source: J. S. House, K. R. Landis, and D. Umberson, "Social Relationships and Health," *Science* 241 (1988): 540–45.

the range of social ties they had—for example, to a spouse, parent, workmate, neighbor, member of a group, and so on. Having given everyone the same measured exposure to infection, he wanted to see which people caught colds (as indicated by all the usual symptoms, such as a runny nose) and whether there were any differences in friendship patterns between those who did and those who did not. Astonishingly, over four times the proportion of people who had fewer social ties developed colds compared with those who had many. This experiment was a refinement and a replication of findings from similar earlier work. Cohen controlled for a great many other variables, including existing levels of antibodies to the virus strains. In subsequent work he has shown that at least some of the difference in infection rates resulted from differences in the functioning of the immune system (Cohen, Doyle, and Skoner 1999).

Research of these different kinds, involving studies of death rates among initially healthy populations, survival after a heart attack, and vulnerability to infections, provides firm evidence that people with better social connections tend to be healthier. There are a number of reviews of the growing body of literature which all confirm the important health benefits of social connectedness (see Berkman and Kawachi 2000; Seeman 2000; Stansfeld 1999).

As if to confirm these patterns, there is now also evidence that *bad* relationships and *bad* marriages are damaging to health. In addition to the long-standing evidence that single and divorced people have worse health than the married, we can now see that bad marital relationships compromise health (Kiecolt-Glaser et al. 1997, 1998; Seeman 2000).

Stress in Early Life

The third of the three most powerful psychosocial influences on health in modern societies is emotional development in early life. A recognition of the processes involved came about in two stages: pre- and postnatal. In a series of studies David Barker showed that birth weight was a predictor of illness at the other end of life—in middle and old age (Barker 1998, 1999). The lower someone's birth weight, the more likely he or she will suffer from conditions such as heart disease, stroke, and diabetes in later life. Initially Barker assumed that low birth weight and its harmful later effects were caused by poor maternal nutrition in pregnancy. He thought the developmental consequences were largely unaffected by later experience. Others thought that low birth weight might simply be a marker for the health effects of socioeconomic deprivation not only at birth but often continuing throughout life. If you experienced more than your share of disadvantage, that would lead to higher rates of disease almost regardless of birth weight. While analyses of data from long-running cohort studies showed there was some truth in the story of continuing disadvantage (Bartley et al. 1994), there were also strong independent effects of birth weight. However, it turns out that in developed countries rather little of the problem of low birth weight is caused by poor nutrition during pregnancy. A study that followed almost seven hundred mothers through pregnancy found no relation between birth weight and intake of any macronutrient at any stage in pregnancy. The only relationship it found with a micronutrient was a beneficial effect of vitamin C in early pregnancy, but the effect was so weak that the authors described it as having "doubtful clinical significance" (Mathews, Yudkin, and Neil 1999). This does not of course mean that poor nutrition in pregnancy can be ignored in countries where nutritional standards are lower. All it means is that in rich developed countries (this population was white women in the south of England) nutritional standards are sufficiently high for poor nutrition not to be an important cause of low birth weight.

What seems to make more difference to birth weight in the developed countries is maternal stress in pregnancy. A study of 2,378 women in Missouri found that mothers of low-birth-weight babies are more likely to give histories of stressful pregnancies (Sable and Wilkinson 2000). There is also evidence that if you stress animals in pregnancy, they have smaller offspring (Drago, Di Leo, and Giardina 1999). Some of the mechanisms connecting maternal stress in pregnancy to low birth weight are now understood. For instance, anxious mothers seem to have reduced uterine blood flow (Teixeira, Fisk, and Gloves 1998). But more important, the link between maternal stress and disease in later life seems to involve levels of stress hormones such as cortisol. Phillips has shown that blood pressure and basal cortisol levels in adulthood are related to birth weight (Phillips et al. 2000; Phillips and Barker 1997). Mothers stressed in pregnancy have higher cortisol levels and there is a strong correlation between maternal and fetal cortisol, which shows that babies are affected by maternal stress before birth (Gitau et al. 1998).

Maternal stress does not just affect health in later life; it leads to important behavioral differences. A study of almost 7,500 children found that maternal stress in pregnancy predicted children's behavior when they were three years old. Children whose mothers were anxious during pregnancy were much more likely than others to develop emotional and behavioral problems (O'Connor et al. 2002). Similar behavioral disturbances of the offspring of stressed mothers have been demonstrated in a wide range of animals (Braastad 1998). One advantage of studying these relationships among animals at the same time as looking at them among humans is that it is possible to use experimental methods with animals that establish the causality of the relationships unambiguously. It has also been possible to demonstrate, at least in rats, that the effects are due to anxiety itself: administering drugs that reduce anxiety "totally counteracted the effects of [experimentally induced prenatal] stress" (Drago et al. 1999).

There is mounting evidence that the effects of prenatal maternal stress are part of a continuum with the effects of stress in infancy and early childhood. Research on the long-term health consequences of social and emotional development from birth into early childhood looks much like the biological side of what psychologists have been telling us for many years about the importance of early childhood. Poor attachment, domestic conflict, loss of a parent—all seem to have lasting effects on physical health.

Research on the long-term health effects of early childhood stress faces two difficulties: the length of follow-up necessary to find the effects and the fact that family life and relationships are a private world into which researchers cannot easily trespass to collect reliable evidence. In the absence of good information about early relationships, researchers have related adult health to more factual things during childhood such as parental death, divorce, or separation, which can be established more reliably and show that relationship problems were likely.

Among the studies which use retrospective accounts of early childhood are a Swedish study of 4,216 people that found that reports of family conflict during one's upbringing was the variable most strongly related to illness in later life after controlling for the father's social class (Lundberg 1993). Coming from "a broken home" was also independently related to later illness. The author concluded by saying, "Social problems stand out as more important for illness later in life than do economic conditions" (1,051). Death rates were over 50 percent higher among people reporting "family dissention" in their family upbringing. In a study of people born in 1946, those whose parents divorced, separated, or died had less good health in adulthood, were more likely to have committed sexual and violent offenses, and were less likely to have good relationships with their own children. The earlier in childhood the family disruption occurred, the stronger the effects (Wadsworth 1984; Wadsworth et al. 1990).

Many studies have shown that people's health is related to their parents' social class independently of the social class they achieved during their adult life (Blane et al. 1996; Gunnell et al. 2003; Davey Smith et al. 1998). That is to say, health is affected by the conditions you experienced in the social class you came from as well as by the class you end up in. A study using psychological measures in adulthood to explore the reasons for this link attributed it primarily to "more unfavorable personality profiles and more negative coping styles" (Bosma, van de Mheen, and Mackenbach 1999: 18). External locus of control, neuroticism, and the absence of "active problem-focused coping" were mentioned in particular. The study concluded by saying, "This finding underlines the importance of psychological mechanisms in the examination of the negative effects of adverse socioeconomic conditions in childhood."

Some researchers who have tended to emphasize the importance of material rather than psychological conditions in childhood have done so because height and leg length (indicating childhood growth) are related to adult health. They assumed that differences in growth were a reflection of nutritional differences, even in rich countries. However, there is abundant evidence that growth is strongly influenced by psychosocial conditions in childhood. Indeed, there is hardly a social worker who would not take failure to thrive as an indication of emotional or physical abuse, and there is a body of literature showing the impact of emotional difficulties on growth, mediated by the impact of psychosocial stress on growth hormone (Albanese et al. 1994; Dykman et al. 2001). Using data from a cohort of 17,000 children born in 1958, Montgomery and colleagues (1997) found that slow growth among seven-year-olds was related to domestic conflict. Similarly, a study of children's growth in German orphanages immediately after World War II, when food was still not plentiful, found that providing extra food in one orphanage was not as important as the contrasting personalities of the matrons in charge (Widdowson 1951). A job transfer in the middle of the experiment revealed that what really helped children's growth was being with a more demonstrative matron instead of a severe one.

Slow growth in childhood not only has psychosocial causes but is also related to psychosocial differences later on. Because of the relationship between growth and psychosocial stress in early childhood, people who are short as children are much less likely to move up the social ladder (Montgomery et al. 1996) and more likely to have higher blood pressure in later life (Montgomery, Berney, and Blane 2000). People who have had a difficult early childhood have a faster rise in blood pressure as they get older, and higher blood pressure in childhood is predictive of higher blood pressure in adulthood (Wadsworth 1991).

Ourselves in the Eyes of Others

Low social status, few friendships, and poor emotional development early in life seem to be the most powerful psychosocial risk factors for less good health in rich countries. Death rates may be two or three times as high among low-status people as among high-status people, and two or three times as high among more isolated people with fewer friends and poorer social networks as among people who are integrated in good social relationships. Nor is there any doubt about the lifelong effects of stress early in life.

However, these risk factors are powerful not only because they are associated with large differences in death rates between those who suffer them and those who don't, but also because such huge numbers of people are exposed to them. Exposure to a toxic chemical at work, or to high levels of nuclear radiation at key sites, may occasionally produce large increases in disease among the exposed, but usually only a tiny proportion of the population is exposed. If we are interested in the main determinants of population health, we need to keep our attention on the risks that are not only powerful but also common.

Low social status, lack of friends, and difficult early emotional development are not the only ways people's lives can go wrong, of course, but they do seem to be the major structural and personal sources of stress to which many specific forms of unhappiness are commonly related. Psychological states such as hostility or depression, a sense of hopelessness, anxiety, and feelings of not being valued have often been shown to fit in closely with the relationship between health and our three primary categories of psychosocial risk. Some of the links are apparent in the psychobiology. For instance, serotonin, which has been described in many species as "the social status hormone," plays an important role in depression. What low social status and depression have in common is low serotonin levels. High-status monkeys not only have higher serotonin levels, but if lower-status animals are given more serotonin, they tend to move up the dominance hierarchy (Raleigh et al. 1991). And modern antidepressants are selective serotonin re-uptake inhibitors, which serve to increase serotonin levels. Kramer has suggested that serotonin, like social status, gives us a feeling of increased security and reduces anxiety, depression, and feelings of self-depreciation (Kramer 1993; Verkes et al. 1998). There are also connections here with friendship. Ob-servations of macaque monkeys showed that higher serotonin levels were also related to greater sociability and more affilia-tive behavior (Mehlman et al. 1995; Higley et al. 1996). An-other interesting biochemical indication that the interactions between the three primary psychosocial risk factors are an important source of many stressful or distressing psychologi-cal states was illustrated by an experiment in which macaque monkeys housed in isolation were found to have low dopamine function (Morgan et al. 2002). When they were put together in social groups, the ones that became high-status showed dramatic increases in dopamine function. Sub-ordinate animals showed no increase in dopamine, despite no longer being isolated. When offered cocaine, which affects similar areas of the brain as dopamine does, the subordinate animals took much more and were more vulnerable to addic-tion.

What is interesting about this picture is how intensely *social* these risk factors are. Whether we look at poor attachment and domestic conflict in early life, low social status, or weak social networks, they are all focused centrally on different aspects of the way we are affected by the quality of social relations.

The biological pathways through which psychosocial risk factors affect physical health and death rates hinge, as we shall see in chapter 8, on the extent to which these risk factors are a source of chronic stress. The most important psychosocial risk factors are the most important sources of stress. This means that what the epidemiological research on psychosocial risk factors has achieved is nothing less than the identification of the most powerful sources of chronic stress in modern societies. This is a very important point to keep in mind—indeed, it is a key to understanding the problematic nature of the social environment in modern societies.

But if we think a little more about these three primary sources of chronic stress, it looks as if they are perhaps pointing to the same central underlying source of stress or anxiety. They are surely all telling us about sources of social insecurity. The personal insecurity that comes from early childhood is connected to the insecurity that can result from low social status. Early stress and the stress of low social status produce many of the same biological, behavioral, and psychological effects. It is not simply that early stress and low status are associated—in monkeys and humans alike—with higher basal cortisol levels, or even that we use similar words (such as insecurity, fears of inadequacy, feelings of inferiority, and anxiety about failure) to describe them. It is also that early insecurity seems to exacerbate, or increase our vulnerability to, the effects of the insecurities that low social status may produce. Indeed, the statistical evidence often shows an interaction between them such that the effects of low birth weight and early insecurity can be substantially offset among children growing up in more advantaged homes (Fraser 1984; Teranishi, Nakagawa, and Marmot 2001; Jefferis, Power, and Hertzman 2002).

The effects of friendship also fit easily into this picture. When you are with friends you feel better about yourself. Friends provide positive feedback: they like to be with you, they enjoy your company, they find you interesting, generous, funny, attractive, or whatever. But if, on the other hand, you feel rejected, if you find yourself having to ask, "Why didn't they invite me?" or "Why doesn't anyone sit next to or talk to me?" you start to doubt whether other people like you. Your confidence drains away; you start to worry that perhaps you are unattractive, boring, gauche, unintelligent, too fat, and so on; the self-doubts and insecurity come crowding in. And, to complete the triangle, how much more vulnerable to these fears are you if you find yourself out of a job or doing something that others around you assume is rather menial?

What these three psychosocial variables—this nexus of intensely social sources of chronic anxiety—is surely pointing to is the way we, as reflexive beings, come to know and experience ourselves through each other's eyes. At the core of what it means to say that, as humans, we are social beings is that we monitor ourselves through each other's eyes. We are tuned into their reactions to us; they are the mirror through which we know and experience ourselves.

This constant monitoring of how others see us is crucial for guiding social behavior and interaction. We need to avoid provoking others to violence against us; we need to solicit their understanding, trust, and cooperation; we need to see when they are surprised, puzzled, amused, or confused by something we have said. Monitoring others' responses to us is also a pre-condition for becoming human beings who are dependent principally on a learned culture rather than on genetically programmed behavior. We acculturate and socialize ourselves through our need to realize ourselves in each other's eyes. Most of what we learn, from our mother-tongue onward, is self-taught and involves imitation, and it is often other people's reactions to us which tell us whether we have got something right or wrong. Other people's perception of us is evaluative and judgmental: they like or dislike, they accept or reject, they trust or don't trust, they look up to or down on us. So essential is this intimate monitoring of others' reactions to us for our security, safety, socialization, and learning that instead of ex-periencing it as their reactions to us, we often experience it as if it were our experience of ourselves. When we do some-thing that is shameful in others' eyes, we can hate ourselves for it, and when we do something that others admire, value, and appreciate, we can get a glowing sense of self-realization.

In an important sense, what we all need is to feel valued. Adam Smith called it the "pursuit of regard." In contempo-rary society we think of people wanting to be respected or loved, either by a small circle just of family and a few friends or, at the other end of the scale, as a celebrity loved by every-one. At the level of the most practical everyday interaction it is the pleasure that comes when we know that something we have done or contributed is appreciated—people enjoyed the meal you cooked, they laughed at your jokes, or they were glad of your practical help, advice, or emotional support. In all sorts of ways we realize ourselves in relation to the needs of others.

Our need to feel valued in others' eyes is sometimes taken

as if it were a mysterious, almost spiritual need. But at bottom it is about security. It is how, in our prehistoric past, we ensured our membership of the cooperative group. Doing things that others found helpful was a source of security: it was our insurance policy that we remained members of the cooperative group, sharing in its benefits and avoiding being outcasts or victimized.

What the epidemiology is surely telling us is that these kinds of anxieties about how others see us—including our worries about being thought unattractive, stupid, ugly, inferior, and the like—are the most powerful source of chronic stress in modern developed societies. Often that becomes focused on whether or not we have friends or on our socioeconomic status in relation to others, and it is deeply colored by early experience. Rising living standards have removed or vastly reduced our worries about meeting basic material needs, keeping a roof over our heads, and where the next meal is coming from, but the increased individualism and geographical and social mobility in modern societies have hugely raised our anxieties about how we appear to others. Where once people lived all their lives in fairly stable communities, we now encounter new people every day. Even over the space of a single decade, surveys have shown increases in the proportion of young people dissatisfied with what they look like—more worried about how they appear to others.

Our reflexivity as human beings, the way we experience ourselves partly through each other's eyes, is close to what many of the great social thinkers from Goffman to Bourdieu, from Heidegger to Fanon, have regarded as the highway through which the social gets into us. No wonder then that it is also the main gateway by which the psychosocial gets under the skin to exert such a powerful influence on health.

The fact that what the epidemiology of psychosocial risk factors is telling us coincides so neatly with the vision of many of the great sociological thinkers should increase our confidence in this interpretation. It represents an important unification of two perspectives, one gained from studies of stress, supported by objective physiological measures, and the other from the perspective of social organization and meaning without regard to biological measures or health indices. It is a triangulation that gives us a fix on the validity of the interpretation.

The Social Emotion?

The psychologist Thomas Scheff (Scheff, Retzinger, and Ryan 1989) called shame *the* social emotion. In his words, "There has been a continuing suggestion in the literature that shame is the primary social emotion, generated by the virtually constant monitoring of the self in relation to others" (Scheff 1990: 79). In his chapter on the physiological display of embarrassment we call blushing, Darwin (1872) argued that shame "depends in all cases on . . . a sensitive regard for the opinion, more particularly the depreciation of others."

Scheff uses the word *shame* as shorthand for a wider range of feelings than we would perhaps normally use the word to describe. He says that when we talk about "having low self-esteem, feeling foolish, stupid, ridiculous, inadequate, defective, incompetent, awkward, exposed, vulnerable, insecure, helpless," we are usually talking about experiences of shame

(Scheff, Retzinger, and Ryan 1989: 181). Many of these feelings are clearly about feelings of inferiority or loss of face in relation to others, and Scheff (1988) describes shame as part of what he calls the "deference-emotion system." Similarly, Gilbert and McGuire (1998) point out, "Shame is nearly always associated with depictions of loss of status . . . of being devalued, disgraced, demoted, and dishonored" (111). Gilbert (1998) has emphasized how feelings of shame result from "processing socially threatening information—particularly in the domains of social rank/status and social exclusions/rejection" (17).

The reason why Scheff calls shame *the* social emotion is because he sees it as the psychological force underpinning both conformity and obedience to authority (Scheff, Retzinger, and Ryan 1989). On the pressure to conform, he discusses Asch's (1952) experiments in which each person around a table was asked to say which of two lines projected on a screen was the same length as a third. All except one of the people were stooges in cahoots with the experimenter and had agreed to give the wrong answer. The point of the experiment was to see what the one naive experimental subject would say when it came to his or her turn to say which of the two lines was equal in length to the third—after everyone else had expressed the same (false) opinion. After these experiments had been repeated a number of times with a succession of subjects, it was found that a large proportion of people tended to conform to the group opinion rather than give an answer which set them apart from others. When asked afterward to explain the answers they had given, people said they feared looking stupid, or thought others would think they "couldn't see straight." But interestingly, some of the people who conformed most appeared to be quite unaware that they had responded to any kind of group pressure.

On the role shame can play in increasing our obedience to authority, Scheff discusses Milgram's (1974) experiments in which people voluntarily administered what they were led to believe were very painful, even life-threatening electric shocks to students in what was presented to them as "a learning experiment." Though they heard what they thought were the screams of their "pupils" in the next room, and often despite clearly feeling worried about what they were being asked to do, many continued to administer shocks when the pupils gave incorrect answers simply because they were instructed to do so by a supervisor. These experiments were set up initially in the 1950s to investigate how human beings had been able to staff and run the death camps in World War II.

The literature on shame is closely related to work on social anxiety, sometimes called social evaluation anxiety. Work on social anxiety links our proneness to feeling shy, and our fear of social evaluation and embarrassment to a wider range of psychological concepts such as fear of negative evaluation, social-evaluative disorder, behavioral inhibition, fear of failure, approval motivation, self-conscious affect, interpersonal competence, self-presentational predicament, sense of inferiority, and inferiority complex, to name but a few. In their different ways these are all concerned with our worries about how we are seen, which inevitably spring from our constant need, as intensely social beings, to monitor how people are reacting to us.

Schore (1998) argues that the shame response develops simultaneously with the growth of the prefrontal cortex of the brain toward the end of the first year of life in the interaction between parent and child following attachment. Soon after the infant has become used to the pleasurable attention and eye contact during the first year, parents start shaping the child's behavior through expressions of disapproval. The suggestion is that the pleasurable face-to-face interactions of attachment are frequently replaced by the caregiver's expressions of disgust. It was because of these early origins that Lewis (1980) called shame the "attachment emotion."

There is, however, widespread agreement that the capacity for shame is innate and that it plays a central role in dominance hierarchies—as the work on obedience to authority suggests. If conflict is to be avoided in dominance hierarchies, dominance has to be matched by submissiveness. As Gilbert and McGuire argue:

> Shame signals (e.g., head down, gaze avoidance, and hiding) are generally regarded as submissive and appeasement displays, designed to de-escalate and/or escape from conflict. Thus, insofar as shame is related to submissiveness and appeasement behaviour, then it is a damage limitation strategy, adopted when continuing in a shameless, nonsubmissive way might provoke very serious attacks or rejections from others. (1998:102)

Leary and Kowalski say, "[W]e favor the idea that social anxiety evolved as a mechanism for fostering social inclusion and minimizing the possibility of rejection or exclusion. . . . The most parsimonious evolutionary explanation of social anxiety is that it evolved as a mechanism for fostering and maintaining one's membership in supportive (i.e. mutually interdependent) groups and relationships." (1995: 27)

Central to these social anxieties are, as we have seen, processes of social comparison and fears of inferiority and inadequacy in relation to others. Trower, Gilbert, and Sherling said that "socially anxious people . . . perceive themselves as subordinates in hostile hierarchies and utilize submissiveness and other 'reverted escape' behaviors to minimize loss of status and rejection" (1990: 39). What Leary and Kowalski describe as the "sociometer theory of self-esteem" links self-esteem, social anxiety, and rejection. Using rather mechanistic terms, they argue that

> the self-esteem system functions as a "sociometer" that monitors the individual's behavior and the social environment (particularly other's reactions) for indications that the person may experience social disapproval or rejection. When cues connoting rejection are detected, the system alerts the individual via negative affect and motivates behavior to restore one's standing with other people. The self-esteem system may have evolved as a mechanism for minimizing the likelihood of social exclusion. (1995: 113)

Feelings of shame do not, however, lead only to timidity and avoidance of conflict. As well as reacting meekly to feelings of shame and accepting one's inferiority, one can reject or contest shame from others. Instead of being conciliatory, one can react to shaming, disrespect, and loss of face with anger and violence. Instead of accepting how others define and see our behavior, violence is often an attempt to avoid loss of face, to reject others' judgment and make them respect us. We shall see more of the role of violence in this context in chapter 5.

Social anxiety is also important in the relationship between friendship and health. In a brief review of numerous studies of social anxiety and social affiliation, Leary and Kowalski say, "People who feel socially anxious tend to disaffiliate" (1995: 157). At its simplest, it is easier to take social initiatives and make friends if you feel confident that you are attractive and will be liked. The empirical research shows that socially anxious people report less contact with friends, have fewer casual conversations, and are less likely to initiate conversations; "socially anxious people who hold negative expectancies regarding the outcomes of interactions have shorter conversations, speak more quietly, and engage in less eye contact with others" (158). Leary and Kowalski point out that this less sociable behavior is a form of avoidance linked specifically to social anxiety. But when facing some nonsocial source of anxiety, even the socially anxious prefer to have friends with them. Nor is it simply that socially anxious people have a lower desire for social contact: the evidence shows that they wish they could participate more fully in social encounters.

Conclusion

We can now see how social anxiety, shame, depression, and violence may all involve evaluative social comparisons and represent various accommodations to, or protests against, perceptions of inferiority, unattractiveness, failure, or rejection. Social status has a direct effect on how others see us, whether boosting pride and esteem or making us feel we are devalued and seen as inferior. Likewise, friendship affects whether you feel rejected or accepted and appreciated, attractive or unattractive, validated in others' eyes or not. And early childhood insecurity influences your behavioral and physiological stress responses throughout life, making people more or less vulnerable to these social anxieties.

Low social status, lack of friends, and early stress are all associated with raised basal cortisol levels and attenuated responses to experimental stressors. We can see why they have been identified in epidemiological studies as the main sources of chronic stress in modern societies. Not only are people who suffer these sources of stress likely to have to live with them for much of their lives, but a large proportion of the population is affected by them.

This, then, is the core of our individual vulnerability to our social environment. Only with a recognition of it can we start to understand which are the important dimensions of the social environment. Without that it is like knowing that someone is allergic to something in the air without knowing what that person is allergic to. Should the person be avoiding pollen, or cats, or dust mites, or what? Knowing not only that it is something in the social environment that we are allergic to but also how our sensitivity works and what aspects of that environment provide the most important triggers means we can go on to see what features of the wider society and social structure may increase or decrease the extent of the problem.

Almost any social problem can be analyzed from an individual or structural vantage point. You can try to identify the individual characteristics that explain which individuals become unemployed, get involved in crime, have problems with drugs, or become depressed. Approaching it in terms of differences between individuals, you are likely to find explanations in people's pasts, their childhoods, their educational experience, their job prospects, and their social networks—or lack of them. But individual characteristics are rarely, if ever, the explanation of why one society has 2 percent unemployment and another 20 percent, or why one society has less than two homicides per hundred thousand population while others have ten times that rate.

If we want to understand why a larger or smaller proportion of the vulnerable run into difficulties, we must understand how the wider economy and social structure damage more people in one society than another. Whether unemployment is 2 percent or 20 percent, homicide rates are high or low, or drug problems are more or less common, it will always be the most vulnerable 2 or 20 percent who succumb. But our knowledge of the nature of how individuals are sensitive to the social environment helps direct our attention to the dimensions of the wider social structure that might make a difference.

4
Health and Inequality
Shorter, Stressful Lives

Measures of Inequality
and Social Status Differentials

In chapter 2 we saw that the quality of social relations—as indicated by levels of trust, violence, and involvement in community life—was better in societies with smaller income differences between rich and poor. In chapter 3 we saw that the quality of social relations and low social status are among the most powerful influences on health. This means that health is likely to be worse in more unequal societies: it will be compromised not only by the bigger burden of low social status and relative deprivation that goes with greater inequality, but also by the poorer quality of social relations in more unequal societies. In this chapter we will see that there is indeed a strong tendency for more unequal societies to have lower average standards of health and shorter life expectancy. Coming at these issues from different angles, the material in chapters 2, 3, and 4 makes a kind of triangulation possible. The consistency between them should give us confidence that we are still closely in touch with reality.

How egalitarian societies are is almost always measured by

the extent of income differences among the population: they tell us whether there are extremes of wealth and poverty in the population, with substantial numbers of very rich and very poor, or whether most people's incomes are bunched closer together nearer the middle. There are a number of common ways of expressing differences in the extent of income inequality; people sometimes use the proportion of a society's total income received by the poorest half of the population. Frequently the poorest half get about 20 percent of the total income in a society while the richest half gets the remaining 80 percent. You could also ask how many times richer the richest 20 percent are than the poorest 20 percent, or what proportion of a society's income would have to be redistributed from the rich to the poor to make everyone's incomes the same. This last is appropriately named the Robin Hood Index. Perhaps the most common measure is called the Gini coefficient. Rather than comparing extremes, it measures the extent of inequality across the whole population and varies between 0 (perfect equality, where everyone gets the same amount) and 1 (perfect inequality, where all income goes to one person). Values for many societies vary around 0.3 or 0.4. Fortunately, although there are so many different measures, they tend to be closely correlated with each other, so the choice of measure usually makes only a small difference to the results of analyses of the relationship between health and inequality across a number of different societies (Kawachi and Kennedy 1997).

An understanding of the effects of inequality on health is particularly relevant to the United States and, to a lesser extent, Britain. As we have already seen, the United States, despite being richer and spending far more per person on medical care than any other country, comes in about twenty-fifth in the international rankings of life expectancy: it performs worse than most other developed countries. The most likely reason for its low health standards is that it is much the most unequal of the developed countries. Britain's position in the international rankings of life expectancy also slipped when income differences widened during the last quarter of the twentieth century.

Before looking at the relation between health and the amount of income inequality in different societies, we should just remind ourselves that health differences between the rich developed countries are no longer related to the *absolute* standard of living and level of income. In chapter 1 we saw how, after the epidemiological transition, the so-called diseases of affluence reversed their social distributions and became the diseases of the poor in affluent societies. Neither among the richest countries nor among the fifty U.S. states is there much evidence of a relation between even twofold differences in real living standards and the life expectancy of the population (Wilkinson 1997; Marmot and Wilkinson 2001). Yet within each of them there are large health inequalities related to relative income and social status. As the effects of absolute poverty have weakened, the social effects of relative deprivation have been unmasked and exposed to attention.

Since I first suggested this interpretation, two research papers following trends in health over time have been published that confirm a tendency for standards of health to lose their association with absolute living standards and become associated with relative standards instead. In 1976 death rates in administrative areas of Taiwan were related to GNP per capita. But in 1995, after life had been transformed by twenty years of extremely rapid economic growth, that relationship had weakened and been replaced by a different pattern. Instead of death rates being lowest in the areas with the highest incomes, it was the areas with the smallest income differences which now had the lowest death rates (Chiang 1999). Similar trends were found in an analysis of changing mortality patterns in the seventeen regions of Spain (Regidor et al. 2003).

In light of the discussion of health risk factors in chapter 3, we should probably think of income distribution in societies as a measure of the extent of social class differentiation among the population. Many research workers in the field interpreted the tendency for standards of health to be related to the scale of income inequality as if it showed us a completely new dimension of influences on health. Instead, it tells us more about the nature of the familiar social class differences in death rates, that relativistic processes situating people in relation to each other are central to social class differences in health and to the social gradient in health.

A possible implication of this is that smaller social class differences may be associated with a shallower social gradient in health—that is, with smaller *absolute* differences in death rates between social classes. Narrower income differences imply that the social hierarchy is less hierarchical and that processes of social class differentiation are weaker. As a result, the number of excess deaths associated with health inequalities could be reduced, and average life expectancy for the society as a whole may be higher.

In well over twenty different independent data sets, involving international analyses as well as analyses of differences between administrative areas within countries, lower death rates have indeed been shown to be related to narrower income differences among populations. (Because some of these data sets have been analyzed by a number of different research workers, there are a much greater number of research papers that report such links.) Against this there are only three or four data sets in which no relationship has been found. In terms of the power of the influences on health, these relationships are particularly important because they deal with the health not simply of small groups exposed to a particular risk, but of whole populations.

Inequality and Health in the United States and Other Rich Countries

Some of the strongest associations between income distribution and health come from analyses of data for areas within the United States. Numerous studies have reported a close relationship between income distribution and age-adjusted death rates in the fifty states (Kennedy, Kawachi, and Prothrow-Stith 1996; Kaplan et al. 1996). Rather like one of the graphs on homicide rates (figure 2.4), figure 4.1 (reproduced from a paper by Nancy Ross and colleagues 2000) includes data for the Canadian provinces as well as the fifty U.S. states. It shows very clearly that it is the most egalitarian states and provinces, rather than the richest, that are healthiest. The fact that average incomes in some states are twice as high as in others is unrelated to death rates. Although the relationships between inequality and health have been shown at all ages, they seem to be strongest among men of working age. Interestingly, this is also the group in which health inequalities are usually found to be largest, suggesting, as one might expect, that income inequality and health inequalities are closely linked.

Figure 4.1: Death rates among men 25 to 64 years old in relation to income inequality in U.S. states and Canadian provinces

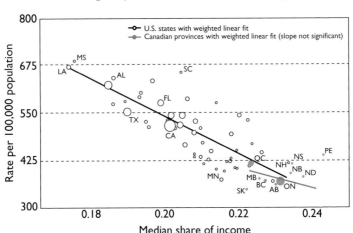

Death rates are lower in U.S. states and Canadian provinces in which income differences are smaller. The measure of income distribution used here is the proportion of societies' total income received by the poorest half of the population. The Canadian provinces are more egalitarian than most U.S. states, so clustering at the lower right end of the distribution.

Source: N. A. Ross, M. C. Wolfson, J. R. Dunn, J. M. Berthelot, G. A. Kaplan, and J. W. Lynch, "Relation Between Income Inequality and Mortality in Canada and in the United States: Cross Sectional Assessment Using Census Data and Vital Statistics," *British Medical Journal* 320 (2000): 898–902. Reprinted with permission of the British Medical Journal Publishing Group.

When this analysis combining data for the U.S. states and Canadian provinces was first published, there was little indication that income inequality was related to the differences in death rates between provinces or cities within Canada. The Canadian provinces all appeared where they should—at the healthier and more egalitarian end of the distribution—but income inequality seemed to tell us nothing about health differences within Canada when considered on its own. More recently this apparent anomaly has been resolved. Inequalities in the distribution of *market* income (that is, income before the deduction of taxes or the addition of benefits) do seem to explain why some Canadian cities are healthier than others (Sanmartin et al. 2003). In addition, an analysis of data for the district health boards in the Canadian province of Saskatchewan has also found that death rates were related to inequality (Veenstra 2002).

The effect of inequality also shows up clearly among American cities. John Lynch and colleagues used data for 282 U.S. metropolitan areas to look at how death rates were related to average income and to income inequality in each city (Lynch et al. 1998). Their results are reproduced in figure 4.2. The height of the columns shows how high the death rates are. Along the right-hand horizontal axis, the cities are arranged into four rows by their average income levels (with a quarter of the cities—about seventy—in each row). The front row of columns shows the death rates in the seventy richest cities, and the back row shows the poorest. Among cities there is a slight tendency for the poorest cities (back row) to have higher death rates, but the really striking pattern is for the more unequal cities (on the left) to have higher death rates than the more equal ones (on the right). On the front horizontal axis the cities are arranged in four categories of income inequality, from the most unequal on the left to the most equal on the right. The scale of the differences in death rates between the tallest column (at the back left) and the shortest (at the front right) is equal to the combined loss of life in 1995 from lung cancer, diabetes, road deaths, human immunodeficiency virus (HIV) infection, suicide, and homicide (Lynch et al. 1998).

**Figure 4.2: Income inequality and mortality in
282 metropolitan areas of the United States**

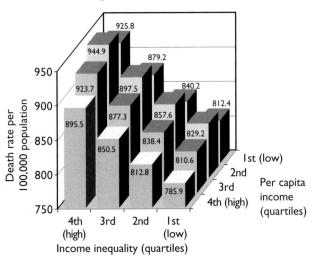

This shows death rates in 282 U.S. cities arranged (along the front) by the amount of income inequality in each, and (from front to back) by the average income in each. The regular steps down from left to right in each row show how much lower death rates are as you move from the less equal to the more equal cities.

Source: J. Lynch, G. A. Kaplan, et al., "Income Inequality and Mortality in Metropolitan Areas of the United States," *American Journal of Public Health* 88 (1998): 1,074–80. Reproduced with permission from the American Public Health Association.

As well as in U.S. states and cities, income inequality and death rates have been found to be related among the counties of Texas (Franzini, Ribble, and Spears 2001) and of North Carolina (Brodish, Massing, and Tyroler 2000). Analyses of zip code areas and census tracts have shown mixed results (Fang et al. 1999; Gorey 1994; Soobader and LeClere 1999). For reasons we shall discuss later, relationships tend to be weaker when inequality is measured in smaller areas: the strongest relationships are found among whole countries, states, and cities; among counties they are often weak and among census tracts often nonexistent.

Going beyond North America, Nancy Ross and Jim Dunn have put together data for some 528 cities in five different countries for which data were available on a comparable basis: the United States, the United Kingdom, Sweden, Canada, and Australia. Figure 4.3 shows that there is a striking tendency for death rates to be higher in cities where there is more inequality. The relationship appears consistent across all the cities, from the most unhealthy and unequal American ones to the healthiest and most egalitarian Swedish and Australian cities. The Australian cities appear to have lower death rates, as befits their level of income inequality, but, like the initial data on the Canadian provinces, inequality does not seem to tell us why some Australian cities are healthier than others. However, the ordering is clear among the U.S. cities considered on their own, as it is among the British cities on their own. Two earlier analyses, using very different methods and data, had shown that income inequality and death rates are related among the 370 or so local government administrative areas of England (Ben-Shlomo, White, and Marmot 1996; Stanistreet, Scott-Samuel, and Bellis 1999).

Also in the developed market democracies obesity has been found to be related to inequality (Pickett et al. forthcoming) and a recent analysis of data for the twenty regions of Italy has found a close relationship between the extent of income inequality and average life expectancy in each region (de Vogli et al. 2004).

Figure 4.3: Income inequality and death rates among working-age men in 528 cities in five countries

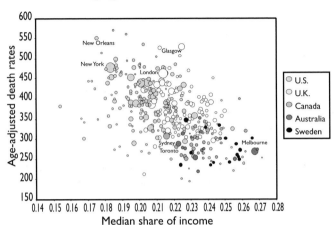

This graph shows that cities in which income differences are smaller tend to have lower death rates. The measure of income distribution used here is the proportion of society's income going to the poorest half of the population, so the more equal cities are to the right. At the most unequal end of the distribution is New Orleans. At the opposite end, with much lower death rates, is Melbourne.

Source: N. Ross, D. Dorling, J. R. Dunn, G. Hendricksson, J. Glover, and J. Lynch, "Metropolitan Income Inequality and Working Age Mortality: A Five Country Analysis Using Comparable Data," *Journal of Urban Health* (in press). Drawn with data kindly provided by Nancy Ross.

Developing Countries

Analyses of international data from both richer and poorer countries have focused particularly on infant mortality. Robert Waldmann, using World Bank data on income inequality from seventy different countries around 1970, found that after controlling for GNP per capita, infant death rates were higher for more unequal countries (Waldmann 1992). This conclusion has been confirmed by Hales and colleagues using more recent data for rich and poor countries (Hales et al. 1999). Figure 4.4, taken from their work, shows that at all levels of economic development infant mortality rates tend to be lower in more egalitarian countries. The figure also shows infant mortality coming down rapidly with increasing GNP per capita among the poorer countries before progressively leveling out among the richer countries. Among the richest countries further economic growth makes little or no difference to mortality.

Figure 4.4: National infant mortality rates in relation to gross national product per head and income distribution

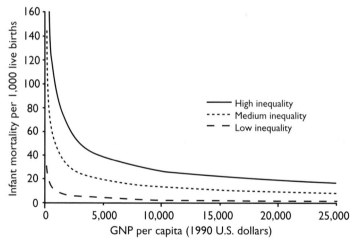

This graph is based on national data from both rich and poor countries. It shows that infant mortality rates decline rapidly as poor countries become richer, but then continue to decline very slowly as countries become much richer. The top curve shows that more unequal countries tend to have higher infant mortality rates at each stage of economic development. The curves below it are for medium- and low-inequality countries.

Source: S. Hales, P. Howden-Chapman, C. Salmond, A. Woodward, and J. Mackenbach, "National Infant Mortality Rates in Relation to Gross National Product and Distribution of Income," *Lancet* 354 (1999): 2,047. Redrawn with permission from Elsevier.

In the earliest of all the analyses of inequality and health, Rodgers found relationships with death rates over a wide range of ages among a group including both richer and poorer countries (Rodgers 1979).

After controlling for GNP per capita, relationships between inequality and infant mortality have been reported among the countries of South America (Casas and Dachs 1998). An analysis of data for the counties of Chile showed that self-rated health was better in counties with smaller income differences (Subramanian et al. 2002). An analysis of data on the condition of schoolchildren's teeth in small areas of the Distrito Federal in Brazil showed that a smaller proportion were decayed, missing, or filled in areas where income differences were smaller (Pattussi et al. 2001).

Communism and the Postcommunist Transition

The early successes and later failures in the health performance of communist countries provides an interesting angle on the relationship between inequality and health. Although many communist countries were once remarkable for the high standards of health they achieved, in many cases standards fell long before the fall of the communist regimes in 1989. Understanding the processes lying behind these changes could tell us a great deal about the changing experience of life in these societies.

A quarter of a century ago, Amartya Sen, who won the Nobel prize for economics in 1998, put together World Bank data for a hundred countries that had a GNP per capita of less than $3,000 in 1977 (Sen 1981). He looked to see how much their life expectancy fell short of eighty years in 1960 and then at the percentage by which they had reduced this short-fall by 1977. Looking at this rate of improvement, he pointed out that nine of the ten countries that had communist governments at the time of his analysis were among the top 25 percent of performers. Among the poorest countries (with a GNP per capita of less than $1,000 in 1977) he found that eight of the twelve that performed best in terms of health improvement were communist. Writing in 1981, he remarked, "Clearly the relative performance of communist countries is superior in terms of this particular indicator" (294). The next group of countries whose performance stood out on Sen's measure were much richer—the "high growth early capitalist countries such as Taiwan, South Korea, Hong Kong and Singapore" (294). Interestingly, a much later World Bank report specifically mentions that all these countries narrowed their income differences between 1960 and 1980 (World Bank 1993). Sen remarks that, in terms of characteristics such as income distribution and poverty reduction, countries from these two groups "have much in common despite their widely different political systems and economic strategies" (1981: 311). Pointing out the power of income distribution and poverty reduction to improve health, Sen calculates that for Sri Lanka to have achieved its high standards of health through economic growth alone, its GNP per capita would have to have been twenty times as high as it actually was.

In the late 1960s life expectancy in a number of the communist countries of Central and Eastern Europe was higher than in some Western European countries, despite what were often very much lower living standards. East Germany outperformed West Germany, and countries like Hungary and Bulgaria also did well. What figures there are suggest that these countries were substantially more egalitarian. Describing the effect of the communist ideology on status systems in Eastern Europe, Swift said:

> [T]he ideological glorification of manual work . . . is, or was, perhaps the most distinctive feature of [social] stratification systems in Eastern Europe. Marxist theory, as filtered through into the official ideologies of societies . . . led manual work to be considered especially important, and non-manual work second-rate. This glorification manifested itself in the prestige system of those societies when compared with those of the West: all research converges on the finding that prestige judgments in the East with respect to the manual and non-manual division were out of line with the rest of the world. Miners, cleaning women, unskilled construction labourers all scored substantially above the standard international metric; government ministers, accountants, office clerks, and lawyers all scored substantially below. (1995: 274)

If the data were available (which they are not), we might expect to find that the relatively good health performance of Eastern European countries up till the late 1960s was rooted in shallower social gradients in health. However, from about 1970, life expectancy ceased to improve and sometimes declined in almost all the communist countries of Eastern Europe despite continued substantial gains in Western Europe (Hertzman, Kelly, and Bobak 1996). By the late 1980s all the Western European countries had higher life expectancy than every Eastern European country.

So why the change? Why did health in a number of Eastern European countries outperform Western European ones up to the late 1960s, only to cease to improve thereafter—so that by the late 1980s they all trailed far behind all Western European countries? The answer is interesting and very pertinent to the present discussion. I have described the socioeconomic changes elsewhere (Wilkinson 1996a) and will only summarize them briefly here. In the late 1960s, the introduction of individual economic incentives associated with the marketization of these societies began to make themselves felt. Two findings show that we are looking at sociological influences on health. First, Clyde Hertzman (1995) showed that the adverse trends could not be explained by factors like air pollution and medical care. Second, and most strikingly, the health trends differ markedly between married and single people. Although married people always tend to have better longevity than single people, the adverse trends in death rates during the 1970s and 1980s were concentrated very largely among single people and led to a dramatic widening of the health gap between married and single people (Hajdu, McKee, and Bojan 1995; Watson 1996). Married people experienced little change in longevity during those years: the downward trend in national figures was very largely due to the deterioration among single people.

Perhaps the best description of what happened was provided by Mikhail Gorbachev when he first became head of state and believed, even at that late stage, that the system could be reformed. His speech to the Central Committee of the Soviet Communist Party on January 27, 1987, was reported in *The Guardian* newspaper (February 2, 1987) as

an extraordinary appeal for the party to renew its social and moral commitment. He spoke of . . . problems . . . which "seriously affected the economy and the social and spiritual spheres." He blamed the party saying "vigorous debates and creative ideas [had] disappeared . . . while authoritarian evaluations and opinions became unquestionable truths. . . . The social goals of the economy in the past few five-year-plan periods were diluted and there emerged a deafness to the social issues. . . . Elements of social corrosion which emerged in the past few years had a negative effect on society's morale, and somehow, unnoticed, eroded the lofty moral values which have always been characteristic of our people. . . . [I]nterest in the affairs of society slackened, manifestations of callousness and scepticism appeared."

The stratum of people, some of them young people, whose ultimate goal in life was material well-being and gain by any means, grew wider. Their cynical stand was acquiring more and more aggressive forms, poisoning the mentality of those around them and triggering a wave of consumerism. The spread of alcohol and drug abuse, and a rise in crime, became indicators of the decline of social mores. Disregard for laws, distortion of reports, bribe taking and the encouragement of toadyism and adulation, had a deleterious influence on the moral atmosphere in society. Real care for people, for the conditions of their life and work and for social well-being, were often replaced with political flirtation—the mass distribution of awards, titles and prizes.

We might now describe these trends as a decline in public spiritedness and social capital. That they are likely to have resulted partly from the economic reforms instituted in these countries by the Soviet Union is suggested not only by their timing, but also by the curious fact that the only country in Eastern Europe where life expectancy went on rising during the 1970s and 1980s was Albania, the only country that, because it adhered to the Chinese Maoist camp rather than the Soviet "revisionist" camp, did not introduce individual economic incentives—perhaps an awkward point for us to digest!

People spoke of the "atomization" of society and the "privatization of social life" during that period (Tarkowska and Tarkowski 1991). This was perhaps the period when the experiment with communism lost its last traces of idealism and the bureaucracies became cynical and self-serving and were seen primarily as agents of Soviet domination. Rises in violence and alcohol consumption provide telltale signs of the adverse trends in the social fabric of these societies.

In 1989–90 these governments were swept aside by a wave of popular opposition. The reforms Gorbachev had hoped to set in motion had failed, and these countries embarked on the difficult transition to market economies. The economic, social, and political chaos that often ensued had devastating effects. Death rates rose rapidly and life expectancy fell catastrophically. The growth of income inequality is probably an indicator of the extent of the disruption and the concomitant growth of both profiteering and unemployment. Death rates in Eastern European countries in 1993 were shown to be related to the extent of their income inequality (Davey Smith and Egger 1996) and, as figure 4.5 shows, even the changes in life expectancy between 1989 and 1995 were found to be closely related ($r = -0.63$) to the changes in income distribution over the same period (Marmot and Bobak 2000). The greater the increases in inequality, the worse the trends in life expectancy.

Figure 4.5: Changes in income distribution and life expectancy: Central and Eastern Europe, 1989–95

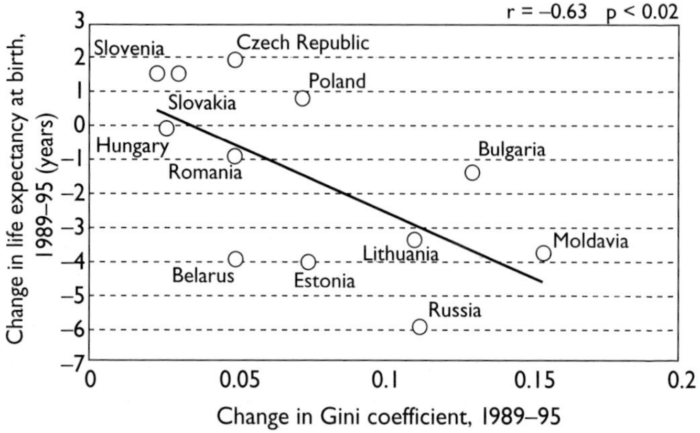

During the economic disruption following 1989, income differences widened through-out the postcommunist countries of Central and Eastern Europe. This graph relates the changes in life expectancy (usually declines) to how much income differences widened during the years 1989–95. The countries at the lower right suffered bigger increases in inequality and bigger falls in life expectancy.

Source: M. Marmot and M. Bobak, "International Comparators and Poverty and Health in Europe," *British Medical Journal* 321 (2000): 1,124–28. Reprinted with permission from the British Medical Journal Publishing Group.

The picture was similar among the eighty-eight regions of the Russian Federation. An analysis of changes in life expectancy during the period 1990–94 found that the rises in death rates had been fastest not in the regions where absolute poverty was greatest, but in those areas where income differences in 1990 were greatest (Walberg et al. 1998). The authors put social cohesion and income inequality at the top of their list of explanations for the decline of life expectancy. They concluded, "These findings add to the growing literature on the complex relation between health, inequalities and social cohesion" (317).

Problems and Anomalies

Though this picture of the relationship between death rates in different societies and the scale of income inequality within them looks strong, there are several data sets that have not shown a relation. Most surprising are analyses that appeared to show no relation between life expectancy and income inequality among the rich developed nations. This was particularly puzzling because it was among the rich countries that I and others initially became aware of this relationship. In 1992 I published a paper showing relationships using three different sets of data for the rich developed societies (Wilkinson 1992). Several other research workers had also shown relationships among the rich countries (Le Grand 1987; Wennemo 1993). In one case it even looked as if the relationship was strong enough to show up what turned out to be anomalies in the data (Wennemo 1993; Wilkinson 1994). These analyses all used data from the 1970s and 1980s. However, later international analyses among the richest countries then found that, with the exception of infant mortality, these relationships had largely disappeared. Relationships between death rates and income inequality got progressively weaker among older people, and actually reversed among the elderly (Lobmayer and Wilkinson 2000). Most recently, however, strong relationships between income distribution and life expectancy among the richest countries have reemerged. Figure 4.6 is reproduced from a paper by Roberto de Vogli and colleagues using data for twenty-one countries (2004).

Figure 4.6: Life expectancy and income distribution in the twenty-one richest countries

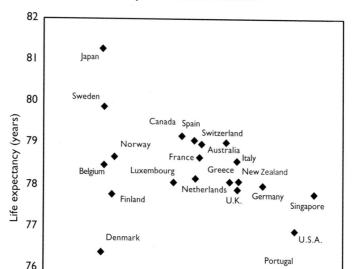

After being disrupted by rapid changes in inequality in the rich countries, the relation between income distribution and life expectancy, apparent earlier, has reemerged. More unequal countries (on the right) tend to have lower life expectancy. When controlled for GNP per capita and weighted by population size, the correlation coefficient r = −0.86.

Source: R. de Vogli, R. Mistry, R. Gnesotto, and G. A. Cornia, "Income Inequality and Life Expectancy: Evidence from Italy," *Journal of Epidemiology and Community Health* (2004); in press. Drawn with data kindly provided by Roberto deVogli.

Why the relationship should have disappeared for a substantial period of time and then reappeared is a mystery. Death rates of older people departed most from what was expected; indeed, relationships between income distribution and infant mortality were never broken. Several other pieces of evidence (too numerous to mention here) showed patterns of death rates at older ages running counter to patterns found at younger ages. It may be that as the main burden of relative poverty moved in many countries from the elderly to families with young children (Kangas and Palme 1998), the elderly were among the beneficiaries of the widening income differences during the 1980s and early 1990s. It is also possible that death rates among the elderly were, for the first time, substantially influenced by medical care, as drugs to control blood pressure and cholesterol levels became widespread. If they had been introduced in some countries before others, the impact of underlying factors such as income distribution would have been masked until their use became widespread in all developed countries. Lastly, the degenerative diseases that dominate mortality in the rich countries reflect lifetime exposure to stress, so death rates at older ages may tend to reflect inequalities of the past and be slow to adapt to more recent changes. This might also explain why infant mortality, which responds faster to current circumstances, continued to reflect income inequality as it changed. However, when it comes to recognizing the impact of inequality on health, the reason this relation was temporarily absent is less important than the fact that the relationship found in data for the 1970s and 1980s has reemerged, as the most recent data (shown in figure 4.6) clearly show.

A large number of studies have now reported empirical relationships between inequality and various health measures. Most of these relationships are statistically too strong to occur by chance alone more than one in a hundred times, or even one in a thousand times. To summarize, we have seen that relationships have been reported among the fifty states and 282 metropolitan areas of the United States, among 528 cities in five developed countries, within cities in Britain and most recently in Canada, among the regions of Russia, in the counties of Chile, and in areas of Brazil, Taiwan, and Italy. In analyses of international data, relationships have been reported several times for infant mortality among both rich and poor countries. Using life expectancy or age-adjusted death rates, relationships have been found both in cross-sectional data and in data showing changes over time among Eastern European countries, as well as separately for Western European countries and among twenty-one rich developed countries.

Several of the studies we have mentioned looked at changes over time rather than just at cross-sectional relationships. We have mentioned the finding that changes in death rates among the regions of Russia during the period 1990–94 were related to the amount of inequality in each at the beginning of that period (Walberg et al. 1998). Rather more impressive is the association shown in figure 4.5 between changes in income distribution and life expectancy in Eastern Europe during the period 1989–95 (Marmot and Bobak 2000). I found a similarly close relationship (see figure 4.7) between changes in *relative* poverty and death rates in European Union countries over the ten years 1985–95 (Wilkinson 1992). In the United States, no clear relationship between changes in income distribution and mortality have been found (Blakely et al. 2000), although the states in which inequality was greatest were found to have the slowest improvements in death rates (Kaplan et al. 1996). However, given that income inequality and death rates do change, and that they do so at different speeds in different countries, cross-sectional relationships between them could only be maintained over time if—whatever the vagaries and time lags—there was some tendency for both sides of the relationship to change together.

Figure 4.7: Annual rate of change of life expectancy in twelve European countries and rate of change in the percentage of the population in relative poverty, 1975–85

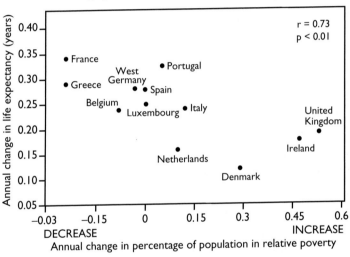

In European Union countries increases in life expectancy were fastest in countries where *relative* poverty declined. (Because of changes in the data series, figures for Portugal are for the second half of the period only.)

Source: Data from M. O'Higgins and S. P. Jenkins, "Poverty in the EC," *Analysing Poverty in the European Community*, edited by R. Teekens and B. M. S. van Praag. (Luxembourg: EUROSTAT, 1990).

Science does not, of course, work simply on the basis of the amount of supportive or contradictory evidence that can be mustered. Most important of all is the ability of a new theory to make accurate predictions of hitherto unobserved facts. In a sense, all the studies conducted since the first time a link between inequality and health was proposed as a general hypothesis should be regarded as tests of it. The data on income inequality and death rates in the fifty U.S. states were first assembled specifically to test the theory that they were related in a context quite separate from the few international analyses that had already been performed. Another analysis, using data for British local authority areas, was also undertaken specifically to test the theory, and in this case I was actually asked before the analysis had been performed whether I would regard this as a fair test. In both instances the results provided confirmation for the theory.

If income distribution and health are related, then there must be a mechanism that links them. From this perspective, the evidence that the quality of social relations is also related to income inequality looks like a successful confirmation of the theory: the quality of social relations is, as we saw in chapter 3, one of the most powerful determinants of health. If health was unaffected by inequality, then presumably the search for a linking mechanism would have proved fruitless. The existence of a strong relation between the quality of social relations and income inequality was unknown to people working in health when the relation between income distribution and health initially came to light. Although there had been many earlier studies of the relation between inequality and violence, they had been published primarily in the criminology journals and were unknown to the few of us thinking about health and inequality. Using largely circumstantial evidence, I had suggested in 1996 that more egalitarian societies scemed more socially cohesive, but the first time this was put to a rigorous statistical test was when Ichiro Kawachi and others looked at the relationship between income inequality and trust among the fifty U.S. states (Kawachi et al. 1997). Not only did they find a very strong correlation ($r = 0.7$), but their statistical analysis of the causal pathway provided strong evidence that the relationship went from income distribution through the quality of the social environment (in this case measured by trust—see figure 2.1) to death rates. Almost the entire relation between income inequality and health was mediated through the quality of social relations.

Other measures of the social environment—besides how much people trust each other—also show that it is indeed the quality of social relations that mediates the relation between income inequality and health. If you use homicides instead of mistrust as an indicator of the quality of the social environment, you get exactly the same result (Wilkinson, Kawachi, and Kennedy 1998). To avoid a circular argument, we subtracted violent deaths from death rates due to all causes to see if the social milieu marked by high rates of violence accounted for the relationship between inequality and higher death rates from all nonviolent causes. Again the answer is yes: only insofar as inequality gives rise to a social milieu characterized by high rates of violence is it related to deaths from all nonviolent causes (Wilkinson et al. 1998). I repeated this analysis (unpublished) with Peter Lobmayer and reached the same conclusions. We also found evidence that the relation between death rates and measures of material deprivation in the counties of England is mediated by the extent of social breakdown consequent on relative deprivation.

As well as the close association between homicides and

other causes of death among the fifty U.S. states ($r = 0.7$), Wilson and Daly (1997) have shown an even closer association ($r = 0.9$) among the seventy-seven neighborhoods of Chicago. The fact that this relationship is close at both the neighborhood and state levels (rather than disappearing at one level after being found at another, as often happens with other factors) strengthens the impression that we are close to the causal processes. The very strong evidence we saw in chapter 2 that homicide is widely and robustly related to inequality is perhaps the strongest evidence that the small differences in inequality between different societies (or between different U.S. states) do indeed have social and behavioral effects.

This statistical confirmation of the causal pathway linking health to inequality suggests that the relationship between them is a causal one. If, against all the odds, the association was just a chance occurrence, we should not expect to find a causal pathway. If the association appeared simply because inequality and death rates were influenced by some other underlying factor, then again, we should not expect to find a plausible causal mechanism running from one to the other. The successful discovery of a mechanism is grounds for confidence that we are in touch with powerful processes impacting on health's sensitivity to the social environment. To explain exactly how these links work, how and why social dominance and inequality drive out sociability, is the task of chapters 5 and 6. Here it is enough to say that because we know both that health is protected by friendship and harmed by low social status, and that more unequal societies are less sociable, it would be surprising if health was not harmed by inequality.

The rest of this chapter deals with some rather technical controversies and may be ignored by more general readers.

The Effect of the Size of the Area Within Which Inequality Is Measured

A famous paper published some years ago in the *New England Journal of Medicine* (McCord and Freeman 1990) showed that death rates in Harlem in New York City were higher at most ages than they were in rural Bangladesh, which is one of the poorest countries in the world. It showed that a boy born in Harlem had less chance of living to age sixty-five than one born in Bangladesh. You might expect that the most important cause of the excess deaths in Harlem would have been violence and drugs, but although death rates were very high from these causes, the most important contributor to these excessively high death rates was heart disease—once again showing the common origins of quite different conditions.

When people first start thinking about inequality as a determinant of health, they often think about social comparisons and imagine that the important social comparisons are between people living in the same neighborhood. This has led a number of researchers to look at inequality within quite small areas. But of course the high death rates in Harlem are not a result of the inequalities *within* Harlem. Rather than being deprived in relation to each other, people in Harlem are deprived primarily in relation to the wider society. It is in relation to the wider society that they come to know their low social status or class position. The social comparisons that define people's class are, by necessity, across classes. This is an important point when thinking about the size of areas over which inequality should be measured. The comparisons have to be over a large enough area to reflect the scale of social stratification between rich and poor. The social comparisons which define class are not those *within* small, socially homogeneous neighborhoods: they involve social class heterogeneity.

Analyses using data for different-sized areas in the United States have shown an interesting pattern. Relationships between health and income inequality tend to be strongest when inequality is measured over large areas such as whole states or cities. At that level we find that the differences in *average* incomes between those states or cities show little or no relation to health. However, if we look at small areas, such as census tracts or zip code areas, the situation is the other way around. Income inequality within these small areas is related weakly, if at all, to health, but the differences in average incomes between the small areas are now closely related to health. Middle-sized areas such as counties show a pattern that falls between the two extremes. Health is moderately related to their average income and moderately related to the inequality within them. Moving from larger to smaller areas results in income inequality becoming less and less important, while differences in average income levels between the areas become more and more important.

What does this tell us? Thinking of the Harlem example, income inequality within Harlem will not pick up the fact that Harlem is deprived in relation to the rest of society, but a glance at the average income in Harlem compared to the rest of the United States will immediately reveal its relative poverty in American society at large. So average income compared to other areas tells us about Harlem's health compared to other areas, but the inequality within it does not.

Social status is determined predominantly within a national framework, and income inequality in the whole nation gives some indication of the depth of the social divisions which have such a profound effect on health. Because of the tendency for people to segregate into rich and poor areas, the smaller the area we look at, the closer we get to something approaching one-class neighborhoods. In most cities there are areas where almost everyone is rich or almost everyone is poor. Differences between the average incomes of these areas becomes more and more important as the indicator of their social status, while inequality within them matters less and less.

Essentially, as we divide large areas into smaller and smaller units, we are converting what was part of the income inequality within the larger area into differences in average income between its smaller constituent areas. At the extreme, we could divide up the large areas into the smallest possible areas—each consisting of just one household. In this limiting case, all the inequality of household incomes in the larger area would have been converted into differences in average income between the single household areas. In effect, by your choice of the size of areas for which you collect data, you can convert income differences between smaller areas into income inequality within larger areas, or vice versa.

The point of going into this in some detail is that there are lots of research papers that ask whether absolute income or income inequality makes the most difference to health. Typically they collect data for small areas to give them plenty of cases for analysis. They then compare whether health is related more closely to inequality within these areas or to the differences in average income between them. Then they assert, with remarkable naiveté, that the income differences between areas are measures of *absolute* income that reflect the direct impact of material conditions on health rather than the effect of relativities between richer and poorer areas. As well as failing to recognize that they could just as well be measures of differences in relative deprivation between each area and the wider society, they also fail to see that if larger areas had been chosen, the differences in average income between the small areas would be converted into income inequality within the larger areas: what were once assumed to be the effects of absolute standards would be converted magically into the effects of inequality! However, the fact that differences in average income or GNP per capita are not strongly related to health in whole countries or states in the developed world is proof that absolute income does not matter.

Rather than being invented as ad hoc attempts to explain away awkward results in small areas, the pattern of stronger association between income inequality and mortality in larger compared to smaller areas was foreseen on the basis of these considerations before most of the data had come in (Wilkinson 1997b). Interestingly, the same tendency for relationships between health and inequality to be stronger when inequality is measured over larger areas was noted (but not explained) in a meta-analysis of studies of the relationship between homicide and inequality (Hsieh and Pugh 1993). This similarity is grounds for increased confidence that the underlying relationships between inequality, on one hand, and either health or violence, on the other, are indeed the same and are likely to involve similar social processes.

Are the Observed Differences in Inequality Large Enough to Matter?

Looking at figure 4.1 (p. 106), which shows the relationship between inequality and health among the U.S. states and Canadian provinces, one might think that the differences in inequality are implausibly small to have such a dramatic impact on death rates. The measure of inequality on the horizontal axis is the proportion of society's total income received by the poorest half of the population. It ranges from just below 18 percent among the more unequal states to around 24 percent in the most equal Canadian provinces. This 6 percent difference might seem too small to have a major impact on death rates. Why should just 6 percent more or less of societies' income, shared between the poorer half of the population, make much difference to anything?

If it was absolute income levels that mattered, that would be a reasonable question, but when we look at it in relative terms things look rather different. Although the differences shown in figure 4.3 (p. 110) are a little larger, let us look more carefully at the 6 percent difference shown in figures 4.1 or 4.3. Table 4.1 shows two societies: a less equal one where the poorest half of the population only gets 18 percent of society's income, and a more equal one where they get 24 percent. The richer half of each society of course gets, respectively, the remaining 82 percent and 76 percent of their society's total income. If, for the sake of argument, the poorer half in each society compare themselves with, or feel their status in relation to, the richest half, then in the less equal society their incomes are $18/82 = 22$ percent of the incomes of the richest half. Similarly, in the more equal society, they are $24/76 = 32$

percent of the incomes of the richest half. So in the less equal
society the poorer half of the population is getting 22 percent
of what they might compare themselves with, and in the
other they are getting 32 percent. The difference between
them, in relative terms, is that the whole of the poorest half of
the population in the more equal society is on average nearly
45 percent better off (32/22) than the poorest half in the less
equal society.

Table 4.1
**Example of income shares of richer and poorer halves of the
population in more and less equal societies**

	Share of income received by poorest 50%	Remaining share of income received by richest 50%	Incomes of poorest 50% as a proportion of incomes of richest 50%
Less equal society	18%	82%	22%
More equal society	24%	76%	32%

So if the richest half of the population set the standards by
which others judge their incomes and/or position in society,
then in relation to them, the average incomes throughout the
whole of the poorest half of the population are 45 percent
higher in the more equal society compared to the less equal
society. In other words, an implausibly small 6 percent difference in shares of absolute income has become a 45 percent
difference in relative income. If we had instead started with
numbers from figure 4.3, varying, say, from 18 to 26 percent
of income going to the poorest half, this calculation would
have produced a 60 percent improvement in the relative posi-

tion of the poorest half of the population. The fact that differences in income distribution that initially appeared to be implausibly small to have much impact on health nevertheless convert to such large differences in the *relative* incomes of the whole of the bottom half of the population is, perhaps, additional evidence that we are right to think in terms of relative income and inequality rather than of absolute income and living standards.

Other Interpretations of the Relationship

People have suggested several ad hoc explanations of the tendency for more egalitarian countries to be healthier. It has, for instance, been suggested that it is a reflection of the ethnic mix of the population or of levels of education. Such explanations suffer from two weaknesses. First, if they work at all, they explain away the relation between income inequality and health in only one or another particular instance in which it occurs, leaving many other examples unexplained. Second, as theories of causality, they fail because, rather than explaining the relationship, they just exchange one explanatory problem for another: instead of explaining why income differences matter, we are left wondering how educational or ethnic differences lower standards of population health.

There is, however, one rival explanation that does have some plausibility and is not limited to a particular context. If death rates were shown to fall faster in response to increases in incomes among the poor than the rich, so that any amount of money did more for the health of the poor than the rich, redistributing income from the rich to the poor might improve average health. This was why I first became interested in the possibility that more equal societies might have better health (Wilkinson 1986, 1992). I had done some research on changing occupational incomes and death rates that showed that any given change in income made more difference to the health of the poor than the rich. The health of the rich was fairly *in*sensitive to changes in income, whereas the health of the poor was—as you might expect—more sensitive to such changes (Wilkinson 1986).

Although that was why I started to look at international data on the relation between income inequality and life expectancy, I soon saw that reducing the health disadvantage of only the poor in each country would not have a big enough effect on overall death rates to explain the inequality association. Despite these origins of the income distribution hypothesis being clearly set out in the initial papers (Wilkinson 1986, 1992), more recent recruits to this field of research have suggested—as if putting forward a novel hypothesis—the possibility that more equal societies might have better health because health was more responsive to income among the poor than the rich (Gravelle 1998)!

What this question boils down to is whether more equal areas are healthier simply because they have fewer poor people (a compositional effect), or whether, over and above that, there is also an effect of inequality itself (a contextual effect) such that people at whatever level of income have lower death rates if they live in a more egalitarian society. The question is, if you allow for the effects of everyone's individual income on their health, is there a contextual effect of inequality on top of that? A number of researchers, usually using data for states or counties in the United States, have looked to see if the association between income inequality and health can be explained by more unequal areas having more poor people, or whether there is a contextual effect of inequality as well. Most find evidence of contextual effects after controlling for individual income, though the smaller the area over which inequality is measured, the weaker the inequality effects (Kennedy et al. 1998; Subramanian, Blakely, and Kawachi 2003; Soobader and LeClere 1999; Subramanian and Kawachi 2004). For reasons we went into above, counties tend to be too small a unit of analysis to pick up more than a small part of the effects of inequality and are therefore an unsuitable basis on which to examine this issue. County-level studies of this issue have therefore come to different conclusions (Mellor and Milyo 2002; Subramanian, Blakely, and Kawachi 2003).

Much the best study of this issue was undertaken by Michael Wolfson, assistant chief statistician at Statistics Canada, the Canadian government statistics agency. To establish the relation between individual income and health in the United States as a whole, he used the National Longitudinal Mortality Study, which, with ten years of follow-up, has 7.6 million person-years of data from a representative sample of the U.S. population. This is the source of the line that curves down throughout its full length from left to right in figure 4.8: it shows the average age-adjusted death rate for people in households at each level of income. The distribution of incomes in the United States as a whole is illustrated by the line that starts off rising and then falls as you move from left to right. It shows that household incomes in 1990 were most frequently around $20,000–30,000 a year but that there was also a long tail of much richer households with incomes over $100,000 a year. Wolfson then used the census to provide data on individual incomes in each of the fifty American states so that he could calculate the death rate you would expect to find in each state on the basis of people's incomes.

Figure 4.8: The distribution of household income in the United States and relative risk of dying at each level of income

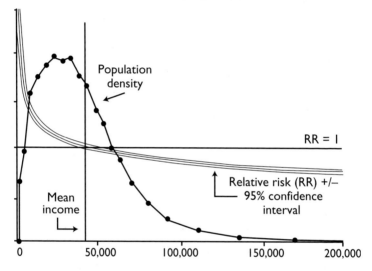

The relationship between household income and relative risk of dying in a given year is shown by the curve declining to the right. The frequency distribution of incomes in the United States, shown by the arched dotted line, tells us how income-related risks of death are distributed in the United States.

Source: M. Wolfson, G. Kaplan, J. Lynch, N. Ross, and E. Backlund, "The Relationship Between Income Inequality and Mortality: An Empirical Demonstration," *British Medical Journal* 319 (1999): 953–55. Reprinted with permission from the British Medical Journal Publishing Group.

Although the findings differ by sex and age, they show that only about one-third of the association between health and inequality can be explained simply by a tendency for more unequal states to have a higher proportion of poor people. The remaining two-thirds of the association between income inequality and health is a contextual effect of inequality on health that raises death rates of people at a given income level if they live in more unequal societies. Figure 4.8 shows why: only a small proportion of people are on incomes low enough to put them on the steeply falling part of the curve relating individual income to death rates. A large majority of the population—all those in households with incomes above about $25,000—are on the gently downward, almost linear (and flatter) part of the relationship. This analysis is the best not only because inequality is measured over large areas (U.S. states), where most of the inequality effects are not lost, but also because the data it uses are based on vast numbers of people and are much more precise than those used in other analyses. Other methods have confirmed this picture (Subramanian, Blakely, and Kawachi 2003).

Not only can the association between health and inequality not be explained away in terms of compositional effects, but the belief that the distinction between compositional and contextual effects is a sensible one to make is based on a misconception. The attempts to make the distinction were initiated by people who clearly thought they were distinguishing between direct material influences on health captured by individual income and some much more mysterious and seemingly implausible *social* or societal effects of inequality itself. They (though not the later defenders of the contextual effect of inequality) assumed that the most important determinants of health were the direct effects of the material goods and services people consume, regardless of the context or standards elsewhere in society. But in chapter 3 we saw the power of psychosocial factors and the reasons for thinking that income within societies is related to health because it marks, as income relative to others, position in the social hierarchy. If we are interested in the effects of inequality and social stratification at the widest level, then to control for individual incomes is overcontrolling—it removes an important component of the contextual effect. To think otherwise is like assuming that each social class is somehow constituted without reference to other classes—as if you can have an upper class without lower classes. It poses the old question, "What is a master without servants?"

There is one more suggested explanation of the effect of inequality we should look at briefly before moving on. John Lynch, its principal proponent, called it "neomaterialism" (Lynch et al. 2000; Marmot and Wilkinson 2001). He coined the term in an attempt to modernize our view of how material circumstances affect health, moving on from the nineteenth-century issues of necessities such as clean water, sewerage, food, and shelter to include things such as cars and home computers as necessary to health.

The suggestion seems to have been motivated less by empirical evidence than by a fear that giving a prominent position to psychosocial pathways would encourage politicians to think that they could forget about the expensive task of reducing poverty and tackle its effects more cheaply by trying to foster better social relations in poor areas. But the truth is exactly the other way around. As we saw in chapter 2, the quality of social relations is powerfully influenced by the scale of income inequality. Rather than the effect on social relations providing a reason for ignoring poverty, it is another major social cost of greater inequality and so an important *additional* reason for tackling poverty.

The neomaterialist approach had several other important weaknesses. Not only did it fly in the face of the evidence that health in the richest countries is related to relative rather than absolute income, but it offered no evidence either that the kinds of consumer goods suggested as neomaterial factors were likely to produce substantial improvements in health or that they mediated the link between inequality and health. Indeed, some of the more prominent items suggested as providing a neomaterial basis for improved health, such as cars and home computers, are just as likely to *harm* health as to protect it—particularly when you think of the combined impact of the sedentary lifestyles that cars encourage, the road deaths, and the effects of increased air and noise pollution.

Part of the neomaterialist view was the idea that greater inequality would lead to a worsening of the educational and material infrastructure in poorer areas, and this would be damaging to health. This suggestion sprang principally from the fact that the structure of local taxation in the United States means that poorer areas lack the tax base to provide adequate funding for their schools and other facilities. But this is primarily an American problem. It does not arise in countries where education has more central funding. In Britain, for example, the Labour Party has political control of most of the major city councils, with the result that city schools actually got more money per pupil than schools in the richer Conservative-controlled rural areas, where councilors were more likely to send their children to private schools. But even in the United States, the argument that inequality might

affect health because of the damage that residential segregation between rich and poor does to the material infrastructure—such as schools in poor areas—is false. Although there
is no doubt that poor areas have worse infrastructure, research
shows that the health effects of inequality are largely independent of residential segregation. An analysis of the health effects of the segregation of rich and poor into separate
residential neighborhoods in 280 U.S. cities showed that although more segregated cities had worse health, segregation
explained very little of the effect of inequality: it was an additional and separate effect (Lobmayer and Wilkinson 2002).

A recent review of the literature on income inequality and
health that ignored all the points made above came to
bizarrely mixed conclusions (Lynch et al. 2004). A travesty of
a review, it made no distinction between data based on larger
or smaller areas, even though the importance of the issue has
been pointed out several times in the research literature and
an earlier review of studies on violence and inequality drew
attention to exactly the same tendency for studies in smaller
areas to produce weaker relationships (Hsieh and Pugh 1993).
Nevertheless, the overwhelming majority of papers showed
clear relationships between income inequality and health. But
rather than reporting this, the associations that were reported
were those remaining after controlling for a host of all the different variables researchers thought fit to try. These included
pathway variables, which should be taken as confirming—
rather than denying—the causal processes; variables that involved overcontrolling; and the ad hoc use of every possible
kind of confounding variable. Controls used in different studies included poverty, income, medical care, welfare transfers,
female labor force participation, illiteracy, alcohol consump-

tion, education, marital status, smoking, household size, race, urbanicity, segregation, unemployment, area deprivation, obesity, social capital, population density, diet, crime, physical activity, and blood pressure.

If we were looking at the effects of economic growth rather than at how unequal and hierarchical a society is, it would be a mistake to control for anything which is likely to be an aspect of economic growth—such as income, ownership of cars or other consumer durables, diet, central heating, proportion of the population employed in manufacturing rather than in agriculture, house size, urbanization, population density, education, etc. If we did control, say, for car ownership, we would not only be removing some of the effects of economic growth, but we would be left looking statistically at only that part of economic growth which was not related to car ownership. The problem with social hierarchy, and so with inequality which serves as its marker, is that social stratification is perhaps the next most fundamental variable to economic development in determining the characteristics of a society. Although its effects are less well understood, they clearly involve the whole social structure and much social behavior, presumably including anything which is patterned by social class. As we saw in chapter 2, Tocqueville started his book *Democracy in America* by making exactly this point about the fundamental influence which "the equality of conditions" has over society. He said he "easily perceived the enormous influence that this *primary fact* exercises on the workings of the society." As he said, "It gives a particular direction to the public mind, a particular turn to the laws, new maxims to those who govern, and particular habits to the governed. . . . [I]ts empire expands over civil society as well as government: it creates opinions, gives rise to sentiments, inspires customs, and modifies everything that it does not produce."

If we think of income inequality as an indicator of the scale of social class differentiation, and we want to see what effect it has on health, then obviously it would be mistaken to control one effect of class differentiation by another. Control variables will reduce the strength of the statistical relation between inequality and health when they are related simultaneously to inequality *and* health. Many are related to inequality simply because social problems and behaviors which, like ill health, are more common in more deprived areas, are likely to increase as greater inequality increases relative deprivation. However, even with the very serious confounding introduced by the use of some controls, the authors of the review classify seventeen of the international studies of inequality and health as providing unqualified support for the relation, eight others as providing no support, and four as having mixed results. If we do the count *before* the use of potentially illegitimate control variables, eighteen of these studies showed a clear link between inequality and health, only four gave no support, and seven gave mixed results. In other words, if we leave out the few studies which had mixed results, over 80 percent of the international studies gave unequivocal support to the link. An even higher proportion of the studies of the *larger* subnational areas, such as regions and metropolitan areas, showed that inequality and health were related, and most did so even after the use of control variables.

Three Final Points

Three points need to be kept in mind when thinking about the evidence of the health effects of inequality presented in this chapter. The first is that the policy implications of the relation between inequality and health are not affected by any of the arguments about how the causal pathways work. From the policy maker's point of view, it makes little difference: redistributing income from rich to poor improves health no matter the mechanism. The second point is that the emphasis placed here on the social environment and psychosocial pathways is of primary relevance only to the rich developed countries well beyond the epidemiological transition. In poorer countries there are obviously also health effects of absolute material standards and levels of consumption—the poorer a country is, the stronger these will be.

The last point is that the relationship between income inequality and health, like the relationship between inequality and the quality of social relations described in chapter 2, is not based on contrasting existing levels of inequality with some unobtainable utopian level of perfect equality. Instead we have confined our attention to the effects of differences in inequality between currently existing nations or regions within nations.

5
Violence and Inequality
Status, Stigma, and Respect

Apart from the first introductory chapter, we have concentrated in chapters 2, 3, and 4 primarily on outlining the basic facts of how people's social relationships and health are affected by the amount of inequality in modern societies. The rest of this book concentrates on explanations of these relationships. In chapter 3 we saw how vulnerable we are as individuals to particular features of the social environment and the way others see us. The most important psychosocial risk factors for health led us to the three most powerful sources of chronic stress in modern societies: stress in early childhood, low social status, and having few friends. These intensely social risk factors affect us by increasing or decreasing our sense of security, making us either more or less at ease with others, more or less worried about how we are seen.

What is at issue here is the difficulty we have, as highly social beings, in negotiating the social world and social relationships. Do we experience other people as a source of support, comfort, and self-realization, or as a source of tension and anxiety putting us on our guard? And how is it that measures of the quality of social relations suggest that greater inequality changes the balance between these two, making social life more difficult? When we understand that, it will then be clear how health also fits into the picture.

Essentially, we should think of the income differences that have provided us with a measure of inequality as indicators of the scale of social class differences in society. Income inequality gives us a rough and ready measure of the size of social distances, of power differentials, of how hierarchical the social structure is, and of how much people are ranked according to what appears as a scale of social superiority and inferiority. In the next two chapters we shall be trying to understand the psychosocial effects of status and class as they impact on people's relations with others and their sense of themselves.

In this chapter we shall show why violence is (as we saw in chapter 2) so consistently more common in societies with larger income differences. In itself, the relationship proves that the differing scale of inequality in different societies has psychosocial and behavioral effects, but we need to understand how the connection works. The relation between violence and inequality provides the best point of entry into understanding the broader social impact of inequality. It will also become clear how violence can be regarded as the extreme case of the pattern of poor social relations associated with inequality.

Why Violence Is Related to Inequality

As we saw in chapter 2, there are now at least fifty papers showing that violence is more common in societies with bigger income differences. This relationship holds up both when we compare different societies internationally and when looking at regions or small areas within them. Already by

1993 there were thirty-four papers, which provided the necessary data to be combined in a meta-analysis, or overview, of the research findings on this relationship (Hsieh and Pugh 1993). The authors concluded that the relation between inequality and violence is robust: all but one of the thirty-seven correlations between a standard measure of income inequality and violence reported in these studies were positive.

In trying to understand the relationship between inequality and violence it is important to recognize that it is not primarily a matter of increased violence between rich and poor. In rare revolutionary situations violence may be more likely to occur between rich and poor, but normally violence is concentrated among the poor themselves: the poorer neighborhoods of most cities are well known to be the most dangerous. Like the statistics on violence, other measures of the quality of social relations also show that relationships tend to be worst in the poorest areas. Using a number of measures of social interaction, including mistrust, Stafford and colleagues (2003) found that the social fabric tends to be worst in the poorest areas. Some researchers have been hesitant to draw attention to this very obvious pattern for fear of being seen as if they were blaming the poor for the problems of poverty, but to deny the effects of low social status prevents us from understanding the powerful force it exerts on its victims. There is a danger of victim-blaming only where people reject a proper situational analysis of the psychosocial effects of low status.

A similar political obstacle to understanding these patterns has been the attempt to deny that violence is more common among the poor by conflating interpersonal physical violence with the institutional violence usually perpetrated by the rich against the poor. Almost by definition, greater inequality means greater institutional violence, benefiting the rich at the expense of the poor. Indeed, Gandhi called poverty the worst form of violence. In a very important sense, what we have to understand is the relation between overt interpersonal violence and the institutional violence of inequality. Lumping both kinds of violence together may seem fairer in apportioning culpability, but—again—it prevents us from understanding the all-important social processes that relate one to the other. We cannot understand one as a response to the other if we make a political principle of not distinguishing between them.

To understand how inequality gets to us and affects whole societies, we need to see how it bears on our social sensitivities. If inequality did simply increase violence between rich and poor, the relationship might seem to need little explanation. But the reason violence between the poor is more common where there is more inequality is more puzzling and understanding it is more illuminating.

Despite the fact that there are so many research papers showing that violence is more common where income differences are larger, there are very few suggestions as to why this is so. But if we look at the literature on violence it is clear that the most frequent trigger to violence is people feeling they are disrespected and threatened with loss of face. Having written on this issue elsewhere (Wilkinson, Kawachi, and Kennedy 1998), what follows provides only a brief summary.

Perhaps the most important academic authority on what leads to violence is James Gilligan. Although he was director of the Center for the Study of Violence at Harvard, to call him merely an "academic authority" does him an injustice. As a prison psychiatrist for twenty-five years, he also saw and talked to violent men almost daily and so has an intimate, firsthand knowledge of his subject. In two books he consistently emphasizes the importance of loss of respect (Gilligan 2001, 1996).

> [T]he prison inmates I work with have told me repeatedly, when I asked them why they had assaulted someone, that it was because "he disrespected me," or "he disrespected my visit" (visitor). The word "disrespect" is so central in the vocabulary, moral value system, and psychodynamics of these chronically violent men that they have abbreviated it into the slang term, "he dis'ed me." (Gilligan 1996: 106)

A few pages later Gilligan goes as far as to say:

> I have yet to see a serious act of violence that was not provoked by the experience of feeling shamed and humiliated, disrespected and ridiculed, and that did not represent the attempt to prevent or undo this "loss of face"—no matter how severe the punishment, even if it includes death. For we misunderstand these men at our peril if we do not realize they mean it literally when they say they would rather kill or mutilate others, be killed or mutilated themselves, than live without pride, dignity and self-respect. They literally prefer death to dishonor. (110)

This is the message above all others that Gilligan conveys. But it is not just the view of a prison psychiatrist or academic. It is also how violence is described by men who have been involved in it themselves. Men such as Nathan McCall (1994) in the United States and Jimmy Boyle (1977) in Scotland have written autobiographies that also emphasize the importance of respect.

Describing street violence in the United States, McCall said:

> For as long as I can remember, black folks have had a serious thing about respect. I guess it's because white people disrespected them so blatantly for so long that blacks viciously protected what little morsels of self-respect they thought they had left. Some of the most brutal battles I saw in the streets stemmed from seemingly petty stuff. . . . But the underlying issue was always respect. You could ask a guy, "Damn, man, why did you bust that dude in the head with a pipe?"
>
> And he might say, "The motherfucka disrespected me!"
>
> That was explanation enough. It wasn't even necessary to explain how the guy had disrespected him. It was universally understood that if a dude got disrespected, he had to do what he had to do.
>
> It's still that way today. Young dudes nowadays call it "dissin'."
>
> They'll kill a nigger for dissin' them. Won't touch a white person, but they'll kill a brother in a heartbeat over a perceived slight. The irony was that white folks constantly disrespected us in ways seen and unseen, and we tolerated it. Most blacks understood that the repercussions were more severe for retaliating against whites than for doing each other in. It was as if black folks were saying, "I can't do much to keep whites from dissin' me, but I damn sure can keep black folks from doing it." (1994: 52)

Jimmy Boyle, who once took pride in being described as the most violent man in Scotland, wrote about status and recognition rather than respect, but the gist of what he says is the same:

There is no doubt that when I was sober, alone and faced with reality I hated myself . . . there was just this completely lost feeling. . . . Yet . . . when I was with my pals, there was this feeling that it was okay and that having attacked a gang single handed the previous night, I had in some way proved myself and gained enough confidence to fight alongside them. I had this hunger to be recognised, to establish a reputation for myself and it acted as an incentive being with the top guys in the district at sixteen. There was this inner compulsion for me to win recognition amongst them. (1977: 79)

Further on in his book Boyle describes a period of fundamental self-examination, and says, "For the first time in my life I was having to think very deeply about violence and other methods of gaining status" (240).

Issues of status and respect become more problematic where there is more inequality. Where income differences are greater, then more people at the bottom are deprived of the money, jobs, housing, cars, and all the things that serve as markers of status and command respect. Without them you are more likely to experience people looking down on you, more likely to become highly sensitive to being regarded as inferior, and increasingly locked into a battle to defend your pride and dignity.

The words of Jimmy Boyle and Nathan McCall fit the picture provided by James Gilligan from the other side of the fence. Together they show how disrespect and wanting status and recognition are part of the struggle against being put down by others, by society at large, against being socially defined as a nonentity, as socially inferior. The struggle for respect is a struggle for human recognition, for social existence itself, and violence is the mother tongue of dominance.

Gilligan mentions cases where prisoners' anxieties about being seen as inferior are linked to feeling deeply ashamed—about being illiterate or about other personal failings. People can feel their lack of status and inferiority to be as visible as if they wore it as a badge of dishonor. As a result, almost any look from someone in even a marginally superior position is likely to be experienced as a negative look—as if it were an immediate perception of the inferiority they feel is written all over them. These feelings can be so strong that rather than wanting recognition, people can aspire to its opposite—invisibility—as the only way to escape from the pain of being defined negatively. Even in middle-class contexts people often say of the experience of shame that they wished "that the ground would just swallow them up," providing them an escape from their embarrassment—often caused by some fairly trivial faux pas. But when in the company of higher-status people, who have more money, education, social know-how, and power, the whole social structure can seem like a conspiracy to define someone as inferior and lacking valued qualities.

The experiential link between the institutional violence of inequality and overt violence on the street was powerfully expressed in the testimony kindly made available to me by Simon Charlesworth (personal communication). It comes from a young man interviewed in Rotherham (a town in the English industrial Midlands), who said:

> Once we leave our neighbourhoods, we're fucked, we're out of our depth, everybody looks an' knows we're like not from there, it's like in Pakistan where they can tell yer from the villages; . . . it's like wi' them who've moved in near me, they're studenty, right middle class, an' I see them lookin' at me, an'

yer thinkin', "Fuck, I don't like them lookin' at me." What it is, thi' do everythin' right—if you ain't got this understandin' everythin' thi' do is right, yer know basically, unless yer see them for what the'r doin'. The'r keepin' themselves to themselves, . . . an' like, if owt [anything] it's us who break the law not them, an' thi' like incite us to do it, the way thi' look at us makes us aggressive, yer feel like yer 'ave to be that way just to get respect, because thi've got the power to do it; it's always gunna be us who's the aggressor against them, not [them] against us, yet the're more violent against us, yer just feel like twattin' them all, know what I mean?

This is a remarkable attempt to describe how apparently harmless behavior, conditioned and informed by status differences, is experienced as close to violence and incitement to violence. The institutional violence that creates the desire for overt violence is nothing more than people appearing to look down from their superior class position. It is experienced as violence against one's social existence: it is the sense of being made to seem inferior that hurts and angers. The anger may seem to have too little cause, but in ordinary social interaction—say, with a friend over dinner at home—we know the danger well enough and are careful to avoid imputations of inferiority to each other—so much so that even if someone said something disparaging about their *own* dress, house, car, intellectual abilities, or whatever, it would be an ordinary kindness to make some remark about their relative merits or to point out offsetting defects of one's own.

The potential for violence between students and other young men described in the quotation above is violence between near equals—between people who may earlier have been equals at the same schools together, but who now have very different destinies. How can we explain why violence is concentrated primarily among the poor rather than between rich and poor?

When I first started trying to understand the effects of inequality I was puzzled by the psychological and sociological literature on social comparisons or relative deprivation, which suggested that, rather than comparing ourselves with people much higher or lower in the social hierarchy than ourselves, we tend to compare ourselves with near equals, with people like ourselves, as if people largely ignored the much larger inequalities above and below them. It was only when reading Robert Sapolsky's *A Primate's Memoir* (2001) that the answer became obvious. Sapolsky described how, among the baboons he watched, conflict tended to be between near neighbors in the dominance hierarchy. The animal ranked number four would conflict with three and five, and the one ranked seventeenth would conflict with sixteen and eighteen. This was clearly because there was no point in fighting animals of a very different rank: the result was a foregone conclusion. For a lower-ranking animal to fight a much higher-status one would be to run a pointless risk for no possible gain. Conflict is concentrated among near equals because it is only between them that relative position is in doubt and rankings can change.

Among humans, near equals can be friends, but we have all heard people say of someone they regard as their equal who seems to be taking on airs or giving any hint of superiority, "Who does she think she is? She's no better than us." Then friendship rapidly turns to anger, because the other person's claim to superiority implies that we are inferior to them. We are watchful of anyone breaking an assumption of equality among apparent equals.

Conflict tends to be concentrated among those lower down in society because the most humiliated feel the greatest need to maintain or regain what McCall described as "what little morsels of self-respect they . . . had left." It is among the most stigmatized, those whose dignity and pride is most damaged by the rest of society, that the fight for dignity can become most demanding. In the quote on page 150 above, McCall also emphasizes the way conflict was—at least in a racial context—concentrated among near equals. After pointing out that blacks largely tolerated the disrespect they got from whites, he said, "It was as if black folks were saying, 'I can't do much to keep whites from dissin' me, but I damn sure can keep black folks from doing it' " (McCall 1994: 52).

Low Social Status and Self-Esteem

The effects of low social status and people's reactions to feeling looked down on have often been regarded as problems of self-esteem. You might well expect that low social status, being poorer than others, or being put down and disrespected, would be damaging to self-esteem. But a review of the accumulated research on self-esteem carried out by Nicholas Elmer (2001) appears to show that there is almost no evidence that they affect it at all. He says that, on balance, the evidence suggests that there is little sign of a social gradient in self-esteem, and noted that African Americans had slightly higher self-esteem than white Americans. He also said the research showed that racists and people involved in violence seem, if anything, to have higher rather than lower self-esteem than others. This not only runs counter to a good deal of popular opinion, but may also seem to conflict with what some might infer from our discussion of the link between violence and inequality.

Elmer's summary of the research seems fair, but the research itself is based on a fatal misconception. We might expect violent people, racists, and people nearer the bottom of the social ladder such as ethnic minorities to have lower self-esteem because—at least in the analysis above—we recognize that they have all suffered from being looked down on. But instead of recognizing the humiliating social processes that are part of social stratification, those privileged to view these problems from above see them simply as if many people lower on the social scale are oversensitive to social status issues—too ready to imagine they are being disrespected or are the objects of racism. Essentially the problem of people feeling put down or treated as inferior is blamed on its victims rather than on its perpetrators and the social structure. It is presented as if the fault lay with their self-esteem rather than with the humiliation they suffer.

But if we do recognize the stigmatizing power of low social status to signify inferiority, how is it that the research seems to show that it doesn't undermine people's self-esteem? Why don't measures of self-esteem show at least something of what we would expect?

To answer this question we have to look at what is going on in a little more detail. The most widely used questionnaire for measuring self-esteem is the Rosenberg Self-Esteem Scale. People are asked how much they agree or disagree with the following ten questions.

1. On the whole I am satisfied with myself.
2. At times I think I am no good at all.
3. I think that I have a number of good qualities.
4. I am unable to do things as well as most other people.
5. I feel I do not have much to be proud of.
6. I certainly feel useless at times.
7. I feel that I am a person of worth, at least on an equal plane with others.
8. I wish I could have more respect for myself.
9. All in all, I am inclined to feel that I am a failure.
10. I take a positive attitude toward myself.

Answering these questions in a way that admits weakness and self-doubt (supposedly revealing low self-esteem) is close to what many people feel they are having to fight against all the time. Questions of this kind may be adequate for looking at some individual differences in self-esteem, but they are insensitive to its social patterning. They fail to recognize that the lower down the social hierarchy people are, the more likely they are to experience life as a continuous challenge to their dignity, and as something that they are constantly having to defend themselves against. Some face what seems almost like a campaign to devalue them. Describing an interview with a particularly violent prisoner, Gilligan says:

> In an attempt to break through that vicious cycle [of violence and punishment] with this man, I finally asked him, "What do you want so badly that you would sacrifice everything else in order to get it?" And he . . . replied with calm assurance, with perfect coherence and even a kind of eloquence: "Pride. Dignity. Self-esteem." And then he went on to say, again more clearly than before: "And I'll kill every mother-fucker in that

cell block if I have to in order to get it! My life ain't worth nothin' if I take somebody disrespectin' me and callin' me punk asshole faggot and goin' Ha! Ha! at me. Life ain't worth livin' if there ain't nothin' worth dyin' for. If you ain't got pride, you got nothin'. That's all you got! I've already got my pride." He explained that the other prisoner was "tryin' to take that away from me. I'm not a total idiot. I'm not a coward. There ain't nothing I can do except snuff him." (1996: 106)

Imagine this man being asked the questions above. In answer to question 7, is he going to say he does not think he is "a person of worth, at least on an equal plane with others"? What would he reply if you asked him if he wished he had "more respect for himself" or whether he thought he failed to take a positive attitude toward himself? You could be fairly sure he would say—with some vehemence—that he is as good as anyone. He might even assert that there is nothing wrong with his self-esteem: as he said, he has his pride, but the problem is that others are trying to take it away from him.

Whatever we think of the psychodynamics involved, we can probably agree that the answers people with this experience of the world might give to questions such as those in the Rosenberg scale may not produce a low self-esteem score: their experience is of having to talk themselves up against a constant barrage of attempts to put them down. Perhaps if we asked people whether they think *others* ignore their good qualities, whether *other people* treat them *as if* they were no good at all, *as if* they have nothing to be proud of, or *as if* they were inferior, the results would come closer to expectations.

Elmer's review of self-esteem research showed that the groups that often came out with marginally higher, rather than lower, self-esteem, were the groups (African Americans, violent men, and racists) who have had their self-esteem challenged and have had to protect themselves from imputations of inferiority linked to low social status. African Americans are less likely to score low on a self-esteem scale both because they recognize the need to resist the injustice of racial prejudice and because of the culture of respect in much of black society. It is, as Nathan McCall (1994) pointed out, because white people disrespected them for so long that blacks have to protect what little self-respect they have left. Violent people are essentially a self-selected group of people who are less willing than most to accept imputations of inferiority. Rather than tolerating being put down, they are prepared to use violence to make people respect them. Finally, the racists, who come out with higher self-esteem than expected, are presumably low-status whites trying to regain their status by downward discrimination: they gain a sense of superiority by rendering others inferior. In short, because people in each of these groups have felt the need to resist society's negative valuation of them, they come out scoring higher on self-esteem scales.

In the present context, the lesson that comes out of Elmer's review of research on self-esteem is that issues of personal value, self-worth, superiority and inferiority, dignity, respect, pride, loss of face, shame, stigma, and humiliation are even more important—and considerably more of a battlefield—than is often recognized. So important is a sense of pride and self-worth that instead of passively succumbing to social definitions of inferiority, we have to defend against them. Sometimes that is merely a psychological defense, and sometimes it involves direct physical attempts to prevent what feel like social assaults. Even those of us who are less likely to be directly involved in violence use other ways of defending ourselves from slights against us—perhaps by pointing out what a pompous idiot the man who made them is. A proper interpretation, then, of the literature on both violence and self-esteem shows not only that self-esteem is so important that it is defended both psychologically and physically, but also that it is inevitably entwined with issues of dignity, personal worth, inferiority and superiority, social status and dominance. After all, "if you ain't got no pride, you ain't got nothin'."

Violence and Shame

Although there is very little psychological literature on the link between violence and *inequality,* there is a good deal on the links between violence and *shame* with which we can fill the gap because, to put it at its simplest, inequality is shaming. Gilbert and McGuire have described how "anger and . . . aggression can substitute for shame" (1998: 23). They say that "covering shame with anger is often referred to as a 'face saving' strategy, known to be a typical source of male violence" (8). Similarly, Thomas Scheff (Scheff, Retzinger, and Ryan 1989) points to the affinity between shame and anger, saying, "[H]ostility can be viewed as an attempt to ward off feelings of humiliation (shame) generated by inept, ineffectual moves, a sense of incompetence, insults, and a lack of power to defend against insults" (188). Indeed, central to his view of the "deference emotion system" is what he calls the "shame-rage spiral" (Scheff 1988: 183). "As humiliation increases, rage and hostility increase proportionally to defend against loss of self-esteem" (188). Anger can be a protective measure to guard against shame, which is experienced as an attack on self. On the relationship between violence, disrespect and social status, Scheff, Retzinger, and Ryan say that "pride and shame states almost always depend on the levels of deference accorded a person: pride arises from deferential treatment by others ('respect'), and shame from lack of deference ('disrespect')" (1989: 184).

Several psychologists and psychoanalysts have suggested that what leads to violence is "unacknowledged shame" (Scheff 1990; Lewis 1980). Rather than having an angry or violent response to some shaming incident, you can of course acknowledge that what you have done is shameful: you can present yourself as shamefaced and apologetic, showing "submissiveness and appeasement behavior"—like a subordinate in a troop of monkeys. But to suggest that the violence that comes when people feel put down and disrespected represents their "failure" to acknowledge shame comes close to saying that people should accept imputations of inferiority. It is surely a mistake to analyze violence without at the same time recognizing the fundamental injustice of class dominance and subordination.

We should not be surprised that although timidity and violence appear to be so different, they are nevertheless linked as alternative responses to status challenges and threats. The shyness and timidity we often feel in the presence of people of higher status are clearly normal expressions of fear that are related to the social evaluation anxiety we discussed in chapter 3. Interestingly, in both Chinese and Japanese, the words for shyness and shame both use the same characters, and in English, the words *anxiety, anguish,* and *anger* all have the same root.

Biological Indicators of Psychological Sensitivity to Social Status

We showed in chapter 3 that low social status was a major source of the chronic stress contributing to class differences in health. There are several biological indicators of our psychological sensitivity to social status differences. For instance, a phenomenon called "white coat hypertension" has long been recognized. It refers to a tendency for blood pressure to be higher when measured by a doctor than when it is monitored electronically or by someone more junior, such as a nurse. It turns out that an important reason why patients tend to be tense with their doctors is that doctors are usually of higher status than their patients. An experiment found that if people are interviewed by someone who is of higher status, their heart rate and blood pressure are higher than if they are interviewed by someone of equal or lower social status (Long et al. 1982). Other psychological experiments have shown that we have a remarkable tendency to assess social dominance ranking even within the first few moments of any interaction (Fisek and Ofshe 1970; Kalma 1991). As Emerson (1883) said, "'Tis very certain that each man carries in his eye the exact indication of his rank in the immense scale of men, and we are always learning to read it."

Psychosocial factors affect health largely through the amount of stress they cause. Stress triggers what we know as the fight-or-flight response. Because the basic processes which have evolved are very old, they are similar among most mammals. As well as mobilizing energy resources ready for muscular exertion, a number of other changes take place, which are outlined in chapter 8. One of these is that levels of a blood clotting factor called fibrinogen increase so that bleeding from wounds stops more quickly. If an animal is stressed because it faces a possible attack and may get wounded, increasing fibrinogen levels obviously make good sense as part of the stress response. Among the nonhuman primates that form social hierarchies—such as baboons, chimpanzees, and macaques—much the most likely threat of attack comes from animals further up the dominance hierarchy. Subordinate animals are frequently attacked and have many more scars and bite marks. Interestingly, the Whitehall II study of civil servants working in government offices in London found that there was a strong social gradient in fibrinogen among both men and women (Brunner et al. 1996). The implication is that the blood of more junior staff clots more quickly. It is as if their bodies were reacting to the stress of subordinate social status by providing protection from physical attack from dominants.

Although higher fibrinogen levels would help limit blood loss in a wounded animal, they also carry an increased risk of heart disease as blood clots can block the coronary arteries. Junior civil servants have four times the death rate from coronary heart disease as their most senior counterparts. Although the differences in fibrinogen are only one of the contributing factors, drugs to thin the blood are very widely prescribed as a preventive measure among older people in the developed world. We could speculate about how much the need for such drugs is a reflection of long-term exposure to stressful social environments in modern societies. Perhaps even the widely beneficial effect of an aspirin a day in reducing heart disease by thinning the blood is an indication that blood-clotting factors in the population at large are undesirably high—as if we were all living under some threat from each other and lacked adequate social support.

A study that specifically compared cardiovascular responses to social stressors with responses to stress from things such as work and financial difficulties concluded, "[I]t appears that conflicts and tensions with other people are by far the most distressing events in daily life in terms of both initial and enduring effects on emotional well-being" (Lassner et al. 1994: 69). The effects of social status differences on blood pressure and blood clotting provide an illustration of how social status gets under the skin. The biological effects of stress associated with social threats have been shown many times. For instance, an experiment in which volunteers were asked to work on math problems (thought to be stressful) initially found no rise in the stress hormone cortisol, but when results were publicly compared with others, there was a clear rise in cortisol levels (Pruessner, Hellhammer, and Kirschbaum 1999). Even children as young as four years old have been found to have raised levels of cortisol in response to shame (Lewis and Ramsay 2002).

We saw (above) that timidity and shyness, despite contrasting sharply with violence, are other possible responses to social status challenges. Depression may be part of the same picture. We might ask why human beings should be so prone to such an incapacitating condition as serious depression. Is it just an evolutionary mistake or can something so apparently dysfunctional have some value? Paul Gilbert (1992) argues persuasively that depression is an evolutionary remnant of a submission response. Dominance hierarchies would lead to continuous conflict if it were not for a capacity to accept subordinate status and submission. If subordinate animals are to avoid dangerous and unwinnable fights, they must recognize their physical inferiority through and through and continuously express themselves as unchallenging. A mind-set consisting of a low self-evaluation, leading depressed people to present themselves as downcast, unchallenging, and unthreatening, could have had survival value if it served to extricate them from unwinnable conflicts.

What lends this perspective particular plausibility is not only that people who study endocrinology among animals sometimes refer to serotonin as the "social status hormone," but also that the drugs used to treat depression are selective serotonin reuptake inhibitors, designed to increase levels of serotonin in the brain. Higher social status among monkeys is associated with higher levels of serotonin, and experiments in which serotonin levels are artificially increased lead to gains in social status (Raleigh et al. 1991; Kramer 1993). There is also some evidence that violent men, whom we might see as resisting being treated or categorized as socially inferior, have higher serotonin than comparable nonviolent men (Moffitt et al. 1998).

Gilbert, a clinical psychologist by profession, lists the various kinds of situations known to cause depression as those in which people feel defeated and devalued and suffer setbacks and loss of control. He also emphasizes that among humans the sense of being defeated, of a failed struggle, does not usually come from involvement with direct social conflict, but may involve a wide range of evaluative domains—everything from insoluble family problems to failure to get promotion at work—in which the depressed person makes "unfavorable judgments about their relative rank, . . . their attractiveness, talents, competencies, desirability to others or 'power.' " As Gilbert says, low self-confidence is affected by unfavorable social comparisons and "can be seen as 'involuntary subordinate self-perception' " (Gilbert and Goss 1996: 25). This fits with Leary and Kowalski's statement that "[t]he most common emotional concomitant of social anxiety is depression" (1995: 137).

Violence is of course much more frequently a feature of male rather than female behavior, and men tend to be more concerned with their status than women are. But an important part of the reason for these characteristics of male behavior is rooted in that fact that, for many women, power, status, and wealth make a man a more attractive sexual partner. Low-status men feel ignored by women who consistently prefer partners able to impress them with signs of money and position. For reasons that I shall describe in chapter 8, circumstances that produce violence in men, particularly young men, produce different responses in women. In the most deprived areas, where rates of violence are highest among young men, teenage pregnancies and depression tend to be high among women. Teenage pregnancies, like violence, are sensitive to inequality (Picket and Wilkinson, forthcoming.) Perhaps one reason why depression is more common among women while violence is more common among men is because in many animal social hierarchies social status has even more important implications for the reproductive performance of males than females. While dominant males attempt to exclude low-status males from breeding, they do not exclude low-status females. So while low-status males had to challenge superiors in order to reproduce, the best strategy for low-status females might be to reproduce while meekly accepting their low status and avoiding the dangers inherent in any challenge.

Perhaps surprisingly, suicide is one of the few causes of death that actually tends internationally to be lower where there is more inequality (McIsaac and Wilkinson 1997; Ng and Bond 2002). Suicide and violence tend to move inversely: in more aggressive societies with more social conflict, people are more likely to blame others when things go wrong, but in societies where the social order is seen as just and has a high degree of moral authority, people are more likely to blame themselves. It is as if, in a more pronounced status hierarchy, people have become more defended against shame in order to maintain their self-esteem against the shame inflicted by low social status. In Harlem, in New York City, suicides were the only important cause of death found to be lower, rather than higher, than elsewhere in the United States (McCord and Freeman 1990). As Durkheim pointed out, some kinds of suicide come from the strength of social relations, from the sense of shame at having let down one's family or work colleagues, while others are more a reflection of isolation and are more likely to be associated, for instance, with unemployment and lack of social connections. It looks as if the predominant pattern varies from country to country, but in most countries (and so in international analyses), perhaps the first is still more important than the second.

6
Cooperation or Conflict?
Inequality Names the Game

What the connection between violence and inequality, described in the last chapter, tells us is that the way in which low social status and relative deprivation get to people most deeply is not through the inconvenience of having to make do with an older car or a less nice house; it is through what having to make do with inferior things says about you. It is the social stigma they carry. They rank you according to your "worth" in comparison to others in society. The implication is that second-rate goods denote second-rate people living second-rate lives: what matters is how what you have compares with others in society. An old car that would be a prized and admired possession in a poorer society is regarded as an embarrassment in a richer one.

Even in late-eighteenth-century England, Adam Smith—usually regarded as the "father" of modern economics—recognized that to be poor feels shameful and thought that this affected minimum acceptable living standards. He said:

> By necessities, I understand not only the commodities which are indispensably necessary for the support of life, but whatever the customs of the country renders it indecent for cred-

itable people, even of the lowest order, to be without. A cred-
itable day labourer would be ashamed to appear in public
without a linen shirt. (1759: 383)

At the other end of the political spectrum, Marx and Engels also recognized the importance of social relativities and
comparisons:

> A house may be large or small; as long as the surrounding
> houses are equally small it satisfies all social demands for a
> dwelling. But if a palace arises beside the little house, the little
> house shrinks to a hovel . . . [and] . . . the dweller will feel
> more and more uncomfortable, dissatisfied and cramped
> within its four walls. (1848: 268)

This underlines the truth of Marshall Sahlins's statement
(quoted in chapter 3) in which he emphasizes that poverty is
not just a small amount of goods, or a relation between means
and ends, but a relation between people, a social status, "an invidious distinction between classes" (1974: 37). If what Smith
and Marx and Engels had to say about the *social* importance of
material differences and "bettering our condition" was true
even before economic growth had rescued the vast majority of
those in the developed world from hunger and the lack of basic
necessities, it must be even truer in the richer countries today.

In recognition of social processes of this kind, poverty in
the European Union is defined as living on less than half the
average national income (or 60 percent of the median), but
some developed countries continue to use absolute poverty
thresholds, which are defined independently of incomes elsewhere in society. We saw in chapter 4 (table 4.1) that although
in absolute terms it might be difficult to see why it should

make much difference whether the poorest half of the population gets 18 or 24 percent of society's income, in relative terms it makes them almost 45 percent better off in relation to the richest half of the population.

Social Corrosion

The link between violence and inequality (chapter 5) testifies to our sensitivity to low social status. It ties together the evidence that the quality of social relations is less good where there is more inequality (chapter 2) to the evidence of our sensitivity to how we are seen and valued by others (chapter 3). We shall now try—as we did with inequality and violence—to make it intuitively clear why more unequal societies are characterized by poorer social relations.

Although homicide is an extreme form of behavior, marking one end of the spectrum of social relations, high homicide rates are (as we discussed in chapter 2) indicative of a more aggressive quality of social relations in society more widely. The following quotation from a twenty-five-year-old man interviewed by Simon Charlesworth in Rotherham describes how the quality of social relations deteriorated in the town as a result of the traumatic decline of local employment in mining and steel.

> [L]ook at it now, it's just gettin' worse an' worse round here. Rotherham's just dog rough now, it's fuckin' dog rough man. All you get . . . is people eyein' yer all time and a lot of 'em aren't hard at all, 'cos hard doesn't have to bother. . . . Who wants to live with every time yer go out of the door some fucker's lookin' at yer? There's this bloke on our street now,

parks his Sierra there and he eyes me out all time. One of these days he's goin' t'catch me in a bad mood and I'm gunna go up and ask him what his problem is. . . . [A]ll these young lads hangin' about on streets acting hard, that's all they've got to do, there's nowt else for 'em to think good about themselves so all they do is attack us, it's us innocent people with families that's sufferin' all time.

You've got to keep yourself fit an' strong, and you've fuckin' got to be able to fight because more an' more now it's comin' down to that 'cos it's the only thing these wankers respect. I mean if they know yer 'andy and they know you've got hard friends . . . X is popular just cos he's fuckin' hard, he's respected and it's all there is for us now. They walk past yer and they stare at yer and first to look away is the weaker one and once they see you as weak, then you're a target to 'em . . . unless they know you've got heavy friends. . . . It's fuckin' rough. (2000: 207)

Among young men, "staring people out" is part of an assertion of status and being "hard" tells people they must respect you and can't take liberties with you. As Daly and Wilson put it: "Men are known by their fellows as 'the sort who can be pushed around' [or] 'the sort who won't take shit,' as people whose word means action or people who are full of hot air, as guys whose girl friends you can chat up with impunity or as guys you won't want to mess with" (1988: 128).

However, the struggle for status and "respectability" has never been confined to the poor. In *The Theory of the Moral Sentiments* Adam Smith recognized not only that the pursuit of what he called "regard" was one of the main driving forces behind economic activity, but also that the accumulation of material wealth was how people gained status. He asked:

[W]hat is the end of avarice and ambition, of the pursuit of wealth, of power, and pre-eminence? Is it to supply the necessities of nature? The wages of the meanest labourer can supply them. . . . What then is the cause of our aversion to his [the labourer's] situation, and why should those who have been educated in the higher ranks of life, regard it as worse than death, to be reduced to live . . . upon the same simple fare with him, . . . and be clothed in the same humble attire? Do they imagine that their stomach is better, or their sleep sounder in a palace than in a cottage? . . . From whence, then, arises that emulation which runs through all the different ranks of men, and what are the advantages [of] . . . that great purpose of human life which we call bettering our condition? To be observed, to be attended to, to be taken notice of with sympathy, complacency, and approbation. . . . The rich man glories in his riches. . . . The poor man, on the contrary, is ashamed of his poverty. (1759: 50)

Powerful modern analyses of the contribution of status considerations to the pressure to consume have recently been provided by Robert Frank in *Luxury Fever* (1999) and by Juliet Schor in *The Overspent American* (1998). Both show the extent to which material consumption is fueled by its power to signify position. Schor shows that the widening income differences in the United States during the 1980s and 1990s led to a rapid increase in the incomes to which people aspired: between the mid-1980s and the mid-1990s surveys show a doubling of the "aspirational" incomes people thought they would need to live as they would like to. The result was that people saved less, spent a higher proportion of their incomes, and were more likely to get into debt—all signs that wider income differences feed into social comparisons and lead to an increasing pressure to consume. Advertisers make the links clear enough.

There is now a growing body of research, much of it nicely summarized by Frank (1999), showing both that people's satisfaction with their incomes is affected by how they compare with others rather than by its absolute level (Clark and Oswald 1996), and that satisfaction and happiness in populations tend to be higher where income differences are smaller (Blanchflower and Oswald 2000, 2003; Layard 2003). As the nineteenth-century philosopher John Stuart Mill put it, "Men do not desire to be rich, but to be richer than other men" (as quoted in Pigou 1932: I.VIII.3).

Social Distancing

One of the nastiest things about dominance hierarchies is the tendency for people to maintain position by asserting superiority over those further down the hierarchy. Indeed, this strategy for maintaining and maximizing rank is a central feature of ranking behavior. George Bernard Shaw expressed it vividly in the *Intelligent Woman's Guide to Socialism, Capitalism and Democracy*:

> The woman from the brick box [i.e., a middle-class woman] maintains her social position by being offensive to the immense number of people whom she considers her inferiors, reserving her civility for the very few who are clinging to her own little ledge on the social precipice; for inequality of income takes the broad, safe, and fertile plain of human society and stands it on edge so that everyone has to cling desperately to her foothold and kick off as many others as she can. (1928: 418)

It would be wrong to quote that without also quoting Shaw's outline, further down the same page, of the alternative strategy:

> There is no word that has more sinister and terrible connotations in our snobbish society than the word promiscuity; but if you exclude its special and absurd use to indicate an imaginary condition of sexual disorder . . . you will see that social promiscuity is the secret of good manners. (418)

Snobbery is one of the ways in which we show, or try to improve, our social status. It is about creating and using distinctions that suggest we are better than those we consider our social inferiors. In previous generations class distinctions were about more than money. Other aspects of culture were used to create and maintain social distances. Just as animals in dominance hierarchies show their physical superiority to each other, so we find symbolic and cultural ways of showing our superiority. In his important book *Distinction: A Social Critique of the Judgement of Taste* (1984), Pierre Bourdieu has demonstrated in a series of surveys the extent to which we use large areas of culture, taste, choice, and aesthetic preference to express social status differences. In general, the upper-class preferences in music, films, art, and books are not simply the more expensive; they are also the less easily appreciated. Social distinctions are consistently marked by a preference for what is less obvious, less accessible, and more exclusive—usually in terms of both content and cost. In comparison with their social superiors, people in lower social groups appear as if they prefer what is more obvious, more sentimental, and less refined. Because aesthetic taste appears as a reflection of one's inner aesthetic sensibilities, differences in taste seem to imply that there are fundamental differences in the way people in different social groups are constituted. They allow people to define themselves as more refined human beings by displaying refined aesthetic sensibilities that seem to speak of the subtlety, refinement, and sophistication of their inner selves. The aesthetics of those at the bottom of society serves to define the "bad" taste that provides the ground against which "good" taste is socially constituted.

So powerful are these processes that to be seen positively, people in lower classes have to avoid socializing where middle-class people predominate and outclass them. Simon Charlesworth describes it like this:

> [T]he lives of working people . . . are based on accommodation to symbolic hierarchies that mark them negatively. . . . They must continually efface the legitimacy of the institutions and manners of the dominant culture. . . . What is characteristic of working class space, therefore, is a suspension of the laws of (cultural) price formation that operate in the fields of the dominant. . . . Thus, the spaces of Rotherham, and especially the leisure spaces—places like the gym, the nightclubs and pubs—are protected markets in which the competence of the people who inhabit those social fields can exist positively, in which the social properties they possess can be said to be capital and not simply a series of deficits. So that within these spaces they can be attractive, charming, eloquent and funny. . . .
>
> Working people thus spend their lives having to pursue a strategy of seeking out spaces in which they can accede to existence in the face of a unified market in symbolic and cultural goods within which their bodily [manner] and speech patterns are hopelessly stigmatised. (2000: 220-21)

In other words, poorer people who want to appear well informed, funny, intelligent, or generous must avoid socializing with better-off, better-educated people who will outclass them, making them appear ignorant, crude, and gauche.

One strategy to avoid being outclassed would be to reduce the differences in behavior and dress, but, as the following quotation from a design student from a poor background shows, that is sometimes more difficult than it seems.

> [T]here's nothin' yer can do, what can yer do: dress smart? If we dress smart they'll spend a load money dressin' down, the'll spend 'undred an' twenty quid on some retro-trainers where we try an' 'ave the best we can afford, we're shown up by tryin' to look smart, thi' can see that money's not there, wi' buy a new jacket an' think wi' got a fuckin' bargain, they spend twice as much on stuff that looks out'r date. (Charlesworth et al. 2004: 57)

Group Density Effect

A phenomenon called the "group density effect" shows how powerfully these processes affect our subjective experience of how we are seen. In a review of research, David Halpern reported that members of minority groups (whether racial, religious, or occupational minorities) tended to have worse mental health if they lived in areas where a *smaller* proportion of the population came from the same minority group. The studies simply take health measures for members of a minority group and correlate them with the proportion of people in their neighborhoods belonging to the same minority. Halpern sums up his review of studies of mental illness by saying:

Taken together, . . . [these] studies constitute extremely strong evidence for some kind of group density effect. . . . Its range and consistency is impressive: it has been reported for religious affiliation, occupational classification, and for numerous ethnic minority groupings. . . . The evidence suggests that, as a general rule, to dwell amongst members of the same perceived group offers some kind of psychological advantage notably manifest in reducing psychiatric admission rates (1993: 605).

What is interesting about these studies is that almost all of the minorities studied are members of disadvantaged groups who usually end up having to live in the poorer areas of our cities. The few members of these minorities doing well enough to live in the better-off neighborhoods, among the majority community, will usually be better off financially and better-educated than other members of the minority group. As a result, they would normally have better physical and mental health than members of the same minority living in the more disadvantaged areas. But a substantial number of studies show that, rather than better health, they have worse health than members of the same minority group who live in the poorer areas where those minorities are concentrated. The health benefits of higher levels of income, education, and social status are being offset by something even more powerful.

The earlier studies (dating from as early as 1939) were all of mental health, and there have been several additions to the literature since Halpern's review was published (see, for instance, Boydell et al. 2001). However, a number of studies have now found the same pattern extends to death rates. In an analysis of heart disease death rates for different ethnic groups in Texas, Franzini and Spears (2003) found that although African American and Hispanics lost more years of life to heart disease than whites, those living in census tracts with a higher density of their own ethnic group lost fewer years of life than their peers living in less segregated tracts. Similar differences in death rates have been found in New York City (Fang et al. 1998). Racial density has also been linked to pregnancy outcomes (Pickett et al. 2005). After controlling for education and marital status, African American women were found to have longer gestations and heavier babies if they lived in richer areas, but only as long as those areas had majority black populations. Pregnancy outcomes of African American women rich enough to live in predominantly white areas bucked this trend: being in a minority offset the advantage of being better off, so birth weights and gestational ages were less good. While a few pieces of research have not confirmed this picture (Karlsen, Nazroo, and Stephenson 2002), the accumulated evidence (which includes studies of the various waves of European immigrants in North American cities) is now strong, if not yet conclusive.

These studies are important because they provide a rare chance to see what happens when the effects of material advantage and of psychosocial processes (in this instance, the effects of feeling you stand out as part of a stigmatized minority) pull in opposite directions. Instead of the normal pattern of social insult being added to economic injury and disadvantage, here people who are *better* off economically end up living in areas where they are likely to feel more constantly aware of their stigmatized minority status. Evidence of a group density effect suggests that the effects of the increased awareness of stigma are more than enough to offset the bene-

fits of higher material standards. Even if part of the health impact of living in areas where there are fewer members of one's
own minority group is caused by a reduction in social support
and friendship networks, that does not make it a fundamentally different phenomenon: that would simply be another
pathway through which the health costs of social divisions
and inequality are incurred.

An interesting confirmation of these same processes can be
found in one of the graphs in Putnam's *Bowling Alone* (2000),
reproduced here as figure 6.1. It shows that in the parts of the
United States where people are less involved in community
life—where, as Putnam has shown, there is more income inequality—it is the poor who have withdrawn from community involvement even more than the rich. Using data for the
fifty U.S. states, figure 6.1 shows that in those states where social capital was weaker, voluntary associations were more
dominated by the better-off. In the low-social-capital states,
the various elected posts in voluntary groups and associations
were even more likely to be held by middle-class people than
they were in the more civic and egalitarian states. What seems
to be happening is that in the areas where income differences
are greater and poorer people are at a greater disadvantage, social prejudices become more apparent and poorer people may
be more likely to worry that these posts are not for them, that
they risk making fools of themselves and may not be wel-
come. Even if they do stand for election, stronger social prejudices may mean they are less likely to be elected.

Given the way we experience ourselves through each
other's eyes and all know the anxiety of negotiating our way
through social space while worrying about whether we are
too fat, too boring, crude, unintelligent, and so on, it is not

Figure 6.1: Social capital and the participation of rich and poor

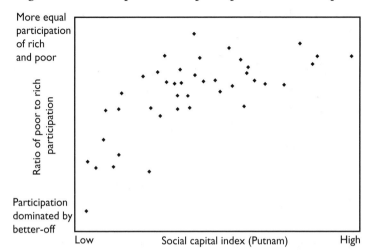

Social capital measures participation in community life, but this graph shows that, in U.S. states, where social capital is lowest (to the left) it is particularly the less well-off who have ceased to participate, and participation in public meetings and associational life is increasingly dominated by the better-off. In states toward the upper right, levels of participation are high and more equally balanced between rich and poor.

Source: Redrawn from R. D. Putnam, *Bowling Alone: The Collapse and Revival of American Community* (New York: Simon & Schuster, 2000), 361, fig. 93. Reprinted with the permission of Simon & Schuster Adult Publishing Group. Copyright © 2000 Robert D. Putnam.

difficult to see how much low social status, or belonging to a stigmatized minority, must increase all these worries. All too easily people can feel out of their league, shown up, and embarrassed. Confidence drains away as we experience our insecurity and feel we lack all the qualities that count.

Dominance Versus Friendship

The empirical evidence suggesting that societies become less friendly as social status differences increase (chapter 2) is not the only link we have seen between social status and friendship. As well as moving inversely in society, social status and friendship also appear linked as important risk factors for poor health. We saw in chapter 3 that friendship was good for health and that lower social status was bad for health. So why are friendship and social status linked strongly in these two quite different ways? Is it just chance that they come together as powerful influences on individual health as well as varying inversely in society?

The answer is that they are not really two completely different variables. They are simply opposite kinds of social relation, like two sides of the same coin. Social status, dominance hierarchies, or animal pecking orders are orderings based on power and coercion. They are fundamentally about gaining privileged access to scarce resources—regardless of the needs of others. In contrast, friendship is based on social obligations, reciprocity, mutuality, sharing, and a recognition of each other's needs. That is why the gift is the symbol of friendship: it says that the giver and receiver do not compete for access to basic necessities. These are simply the two opposite ways human beings can associate: either we come together on the basis of might and who gets what depends on who is strongest and most powerful, or we come together as friends who recognize each other's needs and eschew conflict over access to scarce resources. At bottom, inequality is, as can be seen most clearly among animals, an expression of power relations, and it produces a ranking of people reflecting the differences in their power to gain access to scarce resources.

The reason the difference between relations based on friendship and on social dominance remains so important, why we continue to be so attentive to these dimensions of social life and why they have such powerful implications for chronic stress and health, is rooted in the potential for conflict among members of the same species. The worst rivals faced by members of most species are other members of the same species. Members of different species compete with each other for few if any items, but other members of the same species have all the same needs and want all the same things. As Alexander (1987) put it, the "primary hostile force of nature" (274), which any individual creature has to face, is other members of the same species. As a result, one of the most fundamental problems any species has to deal with is the regulation of competition for scarce resources within the species. Dominance hierarchies and territoriality are just two of the common ways of reducing conflict. Instead of fighting over every scrap of food or every mate, you can avoid a good deal of conflict because status rank makes the result a foregone conclusion for both parties. You back off before being injured rather than afterward. Similarly, although territoriality introduces the burden of defending your territory with regular saber-rattling at the boundaries, it reduces the need to fight over items of food, nesting sites, and mates.

For human beings, as for other animals, our greatest potential competitors are not other species that might compete with us for one or two foodstuffs, but other people. Since we have all the same needs, other people compete with us for everything: food, housing, jobs, sexual partners, the shirt on our backs. But as well as being each other's worst potential rivals, human beings also have an almost unique ability to be each other's best source of assistance, cooperation, comfort, learning, and love. Other people, therefore, have the potential to be our best source of help or most awesome rivals. And whether they are the best or the worst depends on the nature of the relationships between us. Either we compete for access to basic necessities, with the strongest getting the lion's share, or we become friends and agree to share rather than compete. But this is not just an individual issue: different societies work in different ways. Where inequalities are greater, the character of social relations becomes more strongly affected by considerations of power and position, and the processes of social interaction become increasingly infused with the logic of power differentials, dominance, and subordination.

In contrast, equality is the stuff of friendship, reciprocity, and sharing. Both Plato and Aristotle remarked on the incompatibility of inequality and friendship. Plato said, "How correct the old saying is, that 'equality leads to friendship'! It's right enough and it rings true" (1970: 229). Aristotle devoted a good deal of space in his *Ethics* to the difficulties which inequality produces for friendship. He believed that the best forms of friendship could be built only on equality. Few would deny that friendship is more difficult to maintain across great differences in wealth. Differences in material standards give rise to social distances and ideas of superiority and inferiority across which social contact becomes more difficult. So friends tend to be near equals; people tend to marry into their own class—more often the class achieved as a result of education or occupation than class in childhood, if the two differ.

So powerfully do status differences create social distances that we tend to regard the two as almost synonymous. Because bonds of friendship become more difficult across status differences, the team of researchers who put together the Cambridge Scale, for classifying different occupations in hierarchical order of status, based their method on friendship patterns (Prandy 1990). They asked each person in a random sample of the population what was his or her own occupation and what were the occupations of six friends. It was then possible to see which occupations were linked by very few friendships and which were linked by many. The ones linked by many friendships were then considered to be of similar social status and the ones with fewer links to be at a greater social distance from each other. That this method was chosen to derive a hierarchical ordering of occupations, albeit with rather little discussion of the assumptions behind it, shows how firmly embedded—and taken for granted—is the connection between status differences and social distance.

The extent to which friends tend to be near equals is itself an important indicator of how ill at ease we feel with status differences. The difficulty of combining friendship and inequality is of course one of the factors that contribute to the inverse relation between even fairly crude measures of income inequality and the quality of social relations in a society (such as trust, violence, involvement in community life, etc.). But it is only part of the story.

Whether we are related to each other as friends or foes is then a distinction with the deepest psychological roots. The meaning of gift giving and food sharing go to the foundations of human social life. Even now we share food, eat together, and invite friends for a meal because food sharing remains such a powerful social gesture. It symbolizes that we do not compete for the basic necessities of life. Indeed, many evolutionary psychologists argue that the sense of indebtedness, which makes us feel obligated to make a reciprocal gift after having received one, is a human universal (Buss 1999). Giving and accepting the social obligation of reciprocity serves almost as an individual social contract at the foundation of social life. Receiving a gift is to accept a social relation, while to reject one (or even to offer payment for it) is a rejection of a social relation and in some societies is tantamount to a declaration of war.

These ideas around indebtedness and reciprocity go so deep in us that they even lie behind forms of religious sacrifice of the past. Sacrifices are essentially an attempt at gift exchange with the gods: either an attempt to force them to reciprocate by providing good hunting and the like, or a reciprocal gift made after receiving a good harvest or whatever. At the other extreme, the sense of indebtedness is often why bribery works: lavish presents and generosity lead to a sense of indebtedness, which makes it hard for a recipient not to reciprocate by showing favor, albeit corruptly.

The parallel between social and material relations is always close. In warfare each side raids the other's goods without any exchange. And in the closest social relationships, as when a couple gets married or two people start living together, they often combine finances and share resources. Whether we say a society has a nuclear or extended family system is largely a matter of whether or not more distant relatives can call on each other's resources. Right at the heart of our sociality is the problem of how we handle the potential for competition over access to scarce resources. Competition and cooperation are simultaneously material and social relationships. Social and material relationships are mutually defining. Even among nonhuman primates there is evidence that being groomed by another animal creates a social obligation to come to the aid of the groomer when necessary.

At bottom, this is why inequality and dominance relationships go together, why they strengthen or weaken in parallel. Whether the strongest animal in the pack takes its fill before subordinates have a chance or the rich live in sumptuous luxury while the poor go hungry, the message is the same: this is not sharing and reciprocity, this is everyone for him- or herself, and the weakest eat only when there is food to spare.

But inequality and dominance do not only imply the likelihood of material hardship at the bottom. In the primordial setting, systems of dominance and subordination were also systems in which the greater physical strength and aggression of the dominants had to instill matching respect, fear, and submissiveness in subordinates. Those who found themselves in a subordinate position had to have a capacity to fear dominants. As rank provided access to mates, food, comfortable places to sleep, and everything else, rank became a resource in itself. As well as having to be asserted and respected, it also became the mark of fitness, desirability, and superiority—desirability not only in a mate but also in the choice of allies.

Gift Exchange and "Warre"

The same issues come up not simply in relation to the anthropology of the gift or when thinking about dominance hierarchies among nonhuman primates. They are also fundamental to the political thought of philosophers such as Thomas Hobbes. Writing in the English Civil War period in the seventeenth century, Hobbes saw competition between people for necessities as *the* fundamental political problem. As he said:

[I]f any two men desire the same thing, which nevertheless they cannot both enjoy, they become enemies; and . . . endeavour to destroy, or subdue one another. . . . [I]f one plants, sows, builds, or possesse a convenient seat, others may . . . dispossesse, and deprive him, not only of the fruit of his labour, but also of his life, or liberty. And the Invader again is in the like danger of another. (1996: 87)

Hobbes believed people could live in peace only if there was a sovereign power, wielding overriding force and capable of keeping the peace. While "men live without common Power to keep them all in awe, they are in a condition which is called Warre, and such a warre, as is of every man, against everyman" (88). In a "state of nature," before the development of sovereign governments, "every man is enemy to everyman," so life had been, as Hobbes famously imagined, "nasty, brutish and short."

However, Hobbes recognized that even without a governmental power able to keep the peace, societies did not live in an actual state of "warre of each against all": instead they lived with the constant *possibility* of conflict. Talking of conflict between individuals rather than war between nations, Hobbes said:

[W]arre consisteth not in Battell onely, or in the act of fighting, but in the tract of time, wherein the Will to contend by Battell is sufficiently known. . . . So the nature of War, consisteth not in actuall fighting; but in the known disposition thereto, during all the time there is no assurance to the contrary. (88–89)

This theme, the basis of Hobbes's political philosophy, was taken up by Marshall Sahlins in his book *Stone Age Economics*

(1974). He was interested in how the logic of Hobbes's thinking about societies "in a state of nature" related to the actual predominance of gift exchange and food sharing as the bases of exchange relations in hunting and gathering societies. Sahlins argued that the huge social investments people in hunting and gathering societies actually make in each other through gift exchange and food sharing is a response to this constant potential for conflict. He saw the prevalence of gift exchange and food sharing in these societies as an investment in keeping social relations sweet. As he said, "gifts make friends and friends make gifts." The gift amounts almost to a do-it-yourself social contract: it symbolizes a renunciation of competition for scarce resources. Because other people present us with a choice between the benefits of cooperation and the horrors of unlimited conflict, we obviously do all we can to sustain mutually cooperative relations with everyone. And for the same reason, hunting and gathering societies were, as we shall see in chapter 8, highly egalitarian. Only in later forms of society, where we are protected from each other by police forces, can we afford to incur each other's hostility or resentment by amassing private property over which the law guarantees us exclusive rights. One can't help wondering what would happen if the law ceased to protect people's property as soon as its total value exceeded some agreed boundary of social decency while others remained without basic necessities.

It is impossible to read descriptions of the social life of chimpanzees, macaques, or baboons without seeing the common elements in their social hierarchies and ours. Most *modern* class stratification systems may look very different from the displays of power shown by dominant males among some nonhuman primates, but we do not have to look so far back in our history to see human systems where rule was, and sometimes still is, based on naked power and fear. In medieval Europe the feudal nobility often exercised the power of life and death over their serfs and were expected to be personally effective fighters able to lead their troops into battle. Only in the most recent period have substantial parts of the world developed less obviously tyrannical systems. Our tendency to shyness, timidity, and fear in relation to our social superiors, not to mention the tendency for people low in the status hierarchy to have higher blood clotting factors (Brunner et al. 1996), clearly has long evolutionary roots.

With the development of democracy, the long-term trend over recent generations has obviously been for a general softening and decline of authoritarian social stratification systems. If we compare current patterns with our images of the nineteenth century, then whether we look at family relations, relations between employers and employees, relations between social classes, or the way the penal system works, social relations have been mellowing. The use of power is less open and less brutal in all these areas. No longer do parents flog their children. Employees have at least some legal protection from their employers' power. Capital punishment has been abolished in much of the developed world (but not the United States) and is regarded as inconsistent with membership in the European Union.

Somehow all these areas seem to change together. The countries that are particularly advanced in their penal system are also more likely to have better labor laws and employee protection. The same places are more likely to have gentler child care practices and are more likely to have banned teachers and parents from using corporal punishment. The contrast, for instance, between Sweden and parts of the United States is particularly clear. It is not just chance that a failure to abolish capital punishment throughout the United States goes with a failure to develop public services (such as universal access to free medical care) and a failure to provide an adequate social security safety net. Nor is it chance that, among developed countries, the United States has the widest income distribution and Sweden's has historically been among the narrowest.

Much of the softening of social relations over time is clearly predicated on the way economic growth has removed an increasing proportion of the population from absolute want and scarcity. Starvation is no longer the threat it once was. Though we have always had an ability to identify with each other, even to the extent that we flinch involuntarily when we see others hurt, it looks as if we have extended our moral universe so that our ability to identify with others increasingly crosses class and international boundaries that once seemed impermeable, dividing one moral universe from another. Nurtured by gentler early childhoods, aided by more generous material conditions, and perhaps fostered by our daily diet of novels, TV, films, and theater, which encourage us to identify at least with the fictional lives of others, the long-term social trend associated with economic growth has, despite short-term reversals, been toward a gentler and more egalitarian basis of social relations.

However, against this background, there are clearly variations between societies in the progress of our humanity, variations related not only to the level of economic development, but (as we demonstrated in chapters 2 and 4) also to the scale of income differences within societies. Because of the social distances inequalities create, it looks as if they still impose severe limits on our ability to identify with each other.

A Thought Experiment

An important aspect of the interpretation of status and class put forward here is that to understand class we need to think more about our evolution from monkeys than our ideological debt to Marx. What we have been discussing in this chapter is our sensitivity to dominance hierarchies and our social and psychological responses to them. Hierarchies can exist among people and animals alike even in the complete absence of classes based on distinctions such as those between employers and employees or landowners and tenants. But they cannot exist without inequalities in power and access to resources. Dominance hierarchies are fundamentally about using inequalities in power to gain access to resources. On the other hand, if members of a society were divided into classes, each with categorically different relations to the productive system, those differences would become socially and politically charged only if there were inequalities between them giving rise to a perception of the relative superiority of one and inferiority of the other. In other words, it is inequality that gives class its social and psychological power. It is inequality that brings in, or triggers, the psychology of dominance and subordination.

A thought experiment might clarify the relative importance of class and inequality in our own society. Imagine a version of modern market societies in the future. Whether you regard this society as just around the corner or unlikely ever to emerge does not matter. The point is merely to think what a society with the following ground rules would be like. Imagine an advanced market society in which everyone is an employee and dependent solely on earnings. Despite very large income differences, no one receives unearned income or profits: even the people at the top are salaried employees. Although capital markets function much as they do now, all capital is owned by institutions—banks, insurance companies, pension funds, and so on, and the capital belonging to these institutions is traded (much as at present) by employees whose job it is to maximize profits on the stock market. Hence there is no private profit. The top businessmen are as rich as now, but their income comes as a fixed salary rather than from profits. Overall inequality is as large as now, with the same proportions of rich and poor in the population.

The result is a society based on a kind of institutionalized market capitalism in which there is great inequality but no categorical basis for class divisions: no way of dividing distinct classes such as capitalists from workers and landowners from peasants. Everyone is neither more nor less than an employee. The power to hire and fire staff is spread up and down companies, so while people at the top hire and fire senior staff, the poorly paid and poorly educated cleaner close to the bottom is paid 20 percent more an hour than the other cleaners to act as their supervisor, and has the power to hire and fire cleaning staff. My guess is that a society like this, with income inequalities as great as they currently are but with no categorical class divisions, would feel much as our present society does: still the same class prejudices, still the same downward discrimination and snobbishness, still the same problems of relative deprivation and poverty, still the same racial prejudices, still the same experiences of simply being used at work, still the same sense of a system driven by personal ambition and the stock markets' pursuit of profit, just the same injustices of unequal life chances, the same cultural and educational strategies being employed by the better-off to make sure their kids come out on top, and just as much depression, violence, drug use, and kids with educational and behavioral problems—all with the familiar social gradients.

If that is right—and I expect most readers would think it a fair guess that the experience of living in such a society would be all too familiar—then the implication is that it is inequality rather than class that matters. Or to put it differently, inequality and its cultural markers are the essence of the modern class system. Bigger income differences drive bigger status differences, wider divisions, more downward prejudice and discrimination, more "them" and "us," more superiority and inferiority. And, to get back to one of the central subjects of this chapter, that is why it is specifically more *unequal* societies that have less cohesive social relations, and why in concentrating on reducing income inequalities we are not ignoring class (as critics have suggested) but cutting the generative social processes off from the stuff of which modern class divisions are made.

The extent to which the different class divisions of past epochs were determinants of inequality, and how much they were simply the social pegs on which inequality was hung, varied from one society to another. We shall not go into that here. However, no one suggests that different religious, linguistic, or ethnic groups in market democracies are classes. Nevertheless, they are divisions that, when overlaid with inequality, become charged with issues of superiority and inferiority. Tension arises when one group gains a superior social, economic, and political status, and others feel discriminated against and rendered inferior. The subordinate group feels that their dignity is slighted and that they are unjustly treated. Rather than being genuinely structural classes in an economic sense, these kinds of differences merely reflect the social organization of inequality around which the processes of snobbishness and downward discrimination are focused: things such as skin color, religion, language, accent, appearance, and position become socially charged categories when they become markers of status. The same is obviously true where the popular perception of the class divide is the distinction between manual and nonmanual employees or between blue- and white-collar workers. Outward differences take on meaning and become socially charged insofar as they are associated with, and come to stand for, different social statuses. Any outward distinction can become stigmatized and the focus of prejudice where it seems to demarcate the less well-off from the better-off. When such differences are unassociated with social status differences, they are uncoupled from a powerful driver of prejudice and there is usually no inherent reason why they should be divisive and attract discrimination. Indeed, with a high degree of equality across them, they are likely to cause much less friction.

Just as processes of discrimination seek out markers that allow people to be placed in discrete social categories, classes are often imagined as if they were discrete platforms of relative equality in the overall hierarchy of incomes. Almost wherever we are in society, we are aware of people like ourselves, the group of our approximate social equals who seem to be on the same imaginary income platform. We are also aware of people above and below us—presumably on their higher and lower platforms. But a glance at the actual distribution of income shows no sign of platforms, groupings, or discontinuities, just continuous variation (technically close to log-normal).

Social Dominance

If inequality itself is primary, then we need to understand its psychological underpinnings. Social dominance remains such an important sociological issue because of its psychological hold over us.

Jim Sidanius and Felicia Pratto (1999) produced a psychological assessment questionnaire called the Social Dominance Orientation Scale. It measured attitudes toward equality and hierarchy as well as respect for those at the top and prejudice against those below, and it asked a few questions assessing how social or antisocial people's attitudes were—such as whether respondents agreed that "you have to tread on others to get up."

Not surprisingly, this scale was predictive of social attitudes across a wide range of issues. People who scored high on the Social Dominance Orientation Scale were, predictably, more likely to believe what Sidanius and Pratto called the "legitimizing myths" of inequality: they were more likely "to attribute the low incomes of Blacks and Hispanics to things like laziness or lower intellectual ability than to things like bad schools or discrimination" (88). They were more likely than low scorers to oppose "gay and lesbian rights, women's rights, social welfare programmes, mixed race marriages, civil rights policies, affirmative action, immigration." They were also more likely to support "tougher law and order measures, more military expenditure, more money to prisons rather than schools." In short, people "scoring high on SDO were the strongest endorsers of racism, sexism, nationalism, cultural elitism, and patriotism" (84).

Sidanius and Pratto also found predictable differences in scores between people working in "hierarchy enhancing jobs," such as prison guards, police, security officers, prosecutors, and corporate lawyers, who tended to score higher on this scale, and ones in "hierarchy attenuating jobs," such as civil rights and human rights advocates, charity workers, public interest and labor lawyers, social workers, labor organizers, and public defenders, who all scored lower (94).

Sidanius and Pratto regarded themselves as measuring the "universal grammar of social power." They argue that

> the major forms of intergroup conflict, such as racism, classism and patriarchy, are essentially derived from the human predisposition to form and maintain hierarchical and group-based systems of social organization. In essence, social dominance theory presumes that, beneath major and sometimes profound differences between different human societies, there is also a grammar of social power shared by all societies.

To say that this grammar of social power is "shared by all societies" is of course to ignore the very important counterexample of the "assertively egalitarian" hunting and gathering societies that dominated human prehistory (and which we will discuss in chapter 8). But Sidanius and Pratto did test their theories on an impressive number of modern societies across North America, Europe, and Asia.

What is interesting about the Social Dominance Orientation Scale is not so much that you can, for instance, predict people's attitudes toward women's rights from their answers to the social dominance questions, but whether attitudes to social dominance are actually a node around which perceptions of the social world are organized. Is there, in effect, a constellation of social attitudes that move together as one syndrome around some central core that sets the thermostat somewhere on a scale running from dominance and authoritarianism at one end to egalitarian social reciprocity on the other? The Social Dominance Orientation Scale was developed partly to replace measures of the "authoritarian personality"—sometimes called the F scale because it initially came out of attempts to measure fascistic tendencies (Altemeyer 1997, 1998; Adorno et al. 1950).

It was only five years after the end of World War II that Adorno and colleagues published *The Authoritarian Personality* (1950). It was also in the 1950s that Milgram did his experiments (see chapter 3) designed to see if ordinary people would be willing to give what they thought were very painful and dangerous electric shocks to a "learning partner," simply because a white-coated authority figure who seemed to be in charge of the experiment asked them to continue with the experiment (Milgram 1974). It is easy to forget what a shock to psychological thought Nazi Germany and the Holocaust presented. In 1947, John Bowlby, the hugely influential child psychiatrist who developed "attachment theory," said:

> Any organisation, industrial, commercial, national, religious or academic, organised on authoritarian lines must therefore be regarded as inimical to the promotion of good personal re-

lations, of goodness. And that goes for our daily lives . . . in so far as we are authoritarian in our attitude toward others we are promoting bad personal relations and evil. (1947: 39–49)

Work on the authoritarian personality, like the Social Dominance Orientation Scale, involves an integration of thinking about the nature of social relations on the societal and individual psychological levels. Even though the concepts of social dominance and authoritarianism are not the same, they are of course closely related (Altemeyer 1998). They both hinge on the central issue of the conduct of relations with others, and both try to locate people on a continuum of sociability: from the most antisocial interactions, where everything is determined by power, to the mutuality that means we grant equal consideration to each other's needs. Given that social organizations can vary from tyrannical dominance hierarchies to egalitarian systems of reciprocity, the human mind needs to be equipped with the social strategies to make the best of either extreme. The surprise is how finely graded our responses to different amounts of inequality and dominance are.

Before moving on, it is salutary to note that the authoritarian personality scale has been dubbed the "old-fashioned personality scale" (Hartmann 1977; Ray 1990). Essentially, that is a recognition of how fast values were (and perhaps still are) becoming less authoritarian with each passing generation. Not only has it been documented that the ideals of child behavior in the 1920s had much more to do with conformity and obedience to authority than they do now, but there is a clear tendency for older people to score higher on the authoritarian personality scales than younger people. So perhaps we can take comfort from the widespread impression that the historical tide has been moving toward less authoritarian values.

Summary of Links and Direction of Causation

Let us now return to the bones of the argument about the links between inequality and the equality of social relations. Despite the danger of oversimplification, the causal pathways involved are summarized in figure 6.2. The central causal process is the way material differences in living standards are socially distancing: they are read as status differences and so as differences in people's intrinsic merits. Hence, the rich are seen as valued, successful, and significant people, and the poor appear as inadequate failures of little or no account. The difference in living standards are soon fleshed out by cultural differences, which help support perceptions of superiority and inferiority and enable relations between us to be colored by rank. The central role of living standards is expressed in the racist or classist attempt to justify downward prejudice with the assertion that "they just don't live like us."

As inequality increases, we move from strategies favoring cooperative forms of mutual assistance to competitive dominance strategies based on power and aggression. As well-being becomes more dependent on individual material achievement and less dependent on the strength of our social relations, interaction becomes more self-serving and competitive, people trust each other less, they withdraw from social and community activities, and aggression becomes more common. As if social dominance and subordination still gain some of their psychological power from a time when social rank reflected the outcome of trials of strength and aggres-

Figure 6.2: How greater inequality leads to poorer social relations

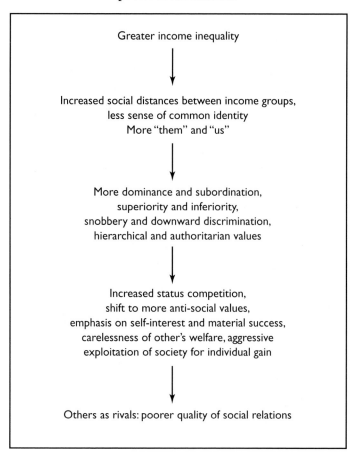

sion, people experience anger, shame, and timidity when at a social disadvantage. The desire to be valued can be satisfied in two different ways: either socially, through the sense of self-realization we get from being active in relation to the needs of others who appreciate what we contribute, or through the more antisocial struggle for the sense of value conferred by higher social status. Both are about validating oneself in the eyes of others, of getting a sense of self-worth. But where one strengthens the bonds of mutual support and affiliation and is more compatible with more egalitarian relationships, the other is divisive, weakens social relations, and is reinforced by the necessity of having to cope with a social structure based on dominance hierarchies in which self-advancement is at a premium.

However, we could look at figure 6.2 and ask whether the relationship from inequality to the quality of social relations might work in the opposite direction from that suggested by the arrows. Do changes in income distribution lead to changes in the quality of social relations, or could changes in the quality of social relations lead to changes in income distribution?

We might note first that changes in income distribution are not usually attributed to changes in social cohesion. More often they are explained in terms of changes in industrial structure, international competition, technology, the demand for different kinds of labor, and other such phenomena. Although few economists would accept that changes in income distribution are primarily determined by changes in the quality of social relations, there are ways in which causality might appear to run from the bottom to the top of figure 6.2. It seems reasonable to expect friendlier, less divided societies, with a strong sense of social justice, to develop narrower income differences. It also seems likely that changes that started in the social relations and ethos of a society could spread to the election of political parties and leaders committed to more or less egalitarian fiscal policies.

But this does not mean we should reverse the direction of the arrows in figure 6.2. Take, for example, the widening of income differences that occurred in many developed countries during the 1980s and 1990s—under Reagan in the United States and under Thatcher in Britain. Many would attribute this major upward shift in inequality to a turning of the ideological and political tide toward the development of neoliberalism, monetarism, and the decline of Keynesian economics.

There is no doubt that neoliberal governments pursued policies that showed little regard for social justice and often weakened the position of vulnerable sections of society. But harming social relations, reducing trust, diminishing involvement in community life, and increasing violence were not the intended outcomes of neoliberal policies. Nor did this new breed of politicians want to increase teenage pregnancies or drug and alcohol abuse, which are other symptoms of social breakdown. If they had foreseen any of these as likely results of their policies, they would have seen them as unintended consequences, or costs, of what they believed needed to be done for other reasons. This means that even if governments pursue policies they know will widen income differences, and their adherence to these policies is partly a reflection of their having less interest in social cohesion, that does not mean that the direction of our causal arrows has been reversed: the unintended social consequences of the widening income differences come about because causality still flows as shown in the diagram, whether policy makers like it or not. Whether their origins were in monetarism and neoliberal policies or what-

ever, widening income differences cannot easily be divorced
from their social consequences. Societies with large income
differences are unlikely to enjoy the quality of social relations
that might be found in much more egalitarian societies. Figure 6.2 may then occasionally operate not with the arrows reversed, but with an arrow looping around from the bottom to
the top, suggesting that there may be feedback effects making
a causal loop or circle, which could turn the whole system
into either a virtuous cycle or a vicious one.

The argument is just the same whether we are considering
government policies that might change income distribution
or a new ethic in the boardroom that leads company directors
to award themselves large pay increases while opposing the
pay demands of their employees. Their actions will also have
divisive social costs.

An important contribution to the link between inequality
and poorer social relations is not included in figure 6.2
(though it is included in figure 1.1 in chapter 1). It involves
the effects of inequality on the stresses and strains of family
life and the impact of that on early childhood. We know that
there is a social gradient in the quality of family social relations (or psychosocial well-being in families): one survey
showed that families living on less than £10,000 a year were
twice as likely to have daily arguments as those with incomes
of more than £20,000 (Relate and Candis 1998). Studies of
marital conflict, domestic violence, maternal depression, children with behavioral problems, and child cortisol levels all
suggest greater stress in poorer families. We also know that
children exposed to domestic violence and/or maternal depression are more likely to be violent in adulthood (most of
the studies are of course of boys). When widening income

differences increase relative poverty, more children will grow up in highly stressed families. In his book *Juvenile Violence in a Winner-Loser Culture,* Oliver James (1995) traced these pathways from the rise in relative poverty in Britain in the 1980s under Thatcher to its effects on children, and subsequently on crime. What this means is that any change in income distribution caused by external economic factors will have powerful lagged effects on the quality of social relations for years to come. The effects of the increase in child poverty that took place in the 1980s and 1990s in a number of countries will leave a permanent mark on the lives and social makeup of a whole generation, affecting their relationships, levels of aggression, and feelings of self-worth or worthlessness.

There are a few examples in which the direction of causality is particularly clear. In chapter 4 we looked briefly at the decline in health and social capital in the Soviet Union and Eastern Europe in the 1970s and 1980s. It is not hard to unravel what causes what. We quoted from the 1987 speech in which Gorbachev, thinking the communist system could still be reformed, drew attention to the decline in standards of public life and came as close as one could in a society based on a centrally planned economy to describing a decline in social capital. He referred to "[e]lements of social corrosion which . . . had a negative effect on society's morale," to a slackening of "interest in the affairs of society," and to "manifestations of callousness and scepticism." At the same time, academic commentators spoke of the "privatisation of social life" during this period (Tarkowska and Tarkowski 1991), and we saw that death rates rose, particularly among single men and women (Hajdu, McKee, and Bojan 1995; Watson 1996), most notably from violence and alcohol-related causes.

Much the most plausible explanation of these adverse social and health trends—which affected all of the former Soviet-bloc countries in Central and Eastern Europe—is that they resulted from the program of economic reforms the Soviet Union pushed on countries in its sphere of influence and which the Chinese opposed and labeled "Soviet revisionism." A response to the earlier uprisings in Eastern Europe, these reforms were designed to gain popular support for the system. At their center was the partial introduction of market mechanisms that included payment systems providing individual economic incentives to employees. An informant interviewed for a T.V. documentary who had been imprisoned after the Hungarian uprising described the reforms as leading to an "atomization" of society (Channel 4 1996). After their implementation, he said, people no longer talked to each other anymore, and the reforms led people to compete with each other for higher standards of consumption. He described how the reforms brought in a new spirit that told people that if they cooperated with the system and worked hard, they would, for instance, not only be able to buy a car, but be able to get a better one than their neighbor's. Though these pressures are familiar enough in Western societies, they seemed to this man a change from the rather more egalitarian, less individualistic, and less competitive society he had known before. In effect, these reforms led to a major increase in competitive consumption.

The very different trends in Albania provide a neat confirmation of this interpretation. As we said in chapter 4, Albania was the only country in Central or Eastern Europe where health standards continued to rise during the 1970s and 1980s and the only country that, because it was allied with China rather than the Soviet Union, did not introduce the program of economic reforms. (It would be wrong to attribute the adverse trends in Eastern Europe to popular opposition to Soviet domination itself: the fact that the same trends were also apparent in the Soviet Union implies that the problem was the policies themselves rather than whether they were self-imposed or imposed by a foreign power.)

This is, then, a story of a decline in social capital caused by economic changes—in this case, changes that dramatically increased economic individualism and widened income differences. The whole story was repeated in the same countries after the collapse of the centrally planned economies in 1989. The rapid widening of income differences during the early 1990s reflected the disruption, dislocation, and insecurity of the economic transition. Death rates rose catastrophically and life expectancy plummeted in many countries, including Russia. Although the rise in heart disease accounted for a larger absolute number of deaths, the percentage rise in violence- and alcohol-related deaths stands out particularly clearly, reflecting, once again, the damage to the social fabric. Several research papers show that the rise in death rates was greatest not where absolute poverty was greatest, as some would expect, but where income differences were widest (Marmot and Bobak 2000; Davey Smith and Egger 1996; Walberg et al. 1998). Once again there can be no doubt of the direction of causality, as economic disruption and dislocation widens income differences and leads to the deterioration of the social fabric and the rise in violence.

There are other examples of change that confirm that social and health changes follow from changes in income distribution. Indeed, there is strong evidence that governments and rulers have always had a sound intuitive understanding of the causal connections between income distribution and social cohesion. There are a number of examples where governments that needed to increase social cohesion and gain popular support introduced more egalitarian policies as a means to this end. The once rapidly growing Asian economies, formerly known as the "Asian tigers," all narrowed their income differences between 1960 and 1980. All eight of them grew rapidly under policies described by the World Bank as "shared growth." A chapter of the World Bank's publication *The East Asian Miracle* (World Bank 1993) described why they became more egalitarian. It says that in all eight of these countries (Japan, South Korea, Taiwan, Singapore, Hong Kong, Thailand, Malaysia, and Indonesia), the governments faced challenges to their legitimacy and needed to gain public approval and support. For instance, South Korea had communist rivals to its north. Taiwan and Hong Kong needed to gain legitimacy in relation to mainland China, and Japan became rapidly more egalitarian after the whole establishment was humiliated by defeat in World War II.

Similar examples can be found in Europe. During World War II, income differences narrowed dramatically in Britain. This was of course partly the effect of war on the economy, which led to a decline in unemployment and a diminution of earnings differentials among employed people. But it was, as we saw in chapter 2, also a result of a deliberate policy pursued by the government to gain the "cooperation of the masses" in the war effort (Titmuss 1958). We quoted from Richard Titmuss's essay "War and Social Policy," in which he says that, to that end, "inequalities had to be reduced and the pyramid of social stratification had to be flattened" (1976: 86).

To ensure that the burden of war was seen as fairly shared, taxes on the rich were sharply increased, necessities were subsidized, luxuries were taxed, and a wide range of food and other goods were rationed to ensure a fair distribution. The Beveridge Report of 1941, which set out plans for the postwar development of the welfare state, including the establishment of the National Health Service, had the same purpose: to present a picture of a fairer future and so gain people's support for the war effort. Although the well-known sense of camaraderie during the war came partly from a sense of unity in the face of a common enemy, it was also increased by the greater emphasis on equality and fairness. If people felt the burden of war had fallen disproportionately on the mass of the working population, leaving the rich unaffected, the sense of camaraderie and cooperation would surely have turned to resentment.

In addition to Britain in World War II and the eight "Asian tiger" countries, some of the earliest welfare state provisions were introduced in the nineteenth century by Bismarck in an attempt to increase social cohesion and gain popular support for his political program of unifying the separate German states.

A much smaller scale example of economic change leading to changes in social relations comes from Charlesworth's (2000) study showing how life in Rotherham changed following a decline in employment in the mining and steel industries on which the town had been dependent. Before the loss of employment, it had, like other mining communities, a fairly coherent social life. But as unemployment rose, the quality of social interaction on the streets, particularly among younger people, became increasingly aggressive and antisocial. In chapter 5 we saw a typical complaint of a local who, very much aware of the social changes going on around him, described people as becoming "hard" and the place as getting "dog rough." He said you have to keep yourself "fit and strong . . . to be able to fight because more an' more now it's comin' down to that." This is very much like descriptions of what has happened to the social fabric in other mining areas, such as the Welsh valleys, which suffered steep rises in unemployment as coal mining declined under Thatcher. There is the same cult of being "hard" and a huge rise in drug abuse. Once again, the social changes clearly follow from the economic ones.

A very different example of the link between inequality and the quality of social relations that provides another opportunity to see how causality might have worked comes from the small Italian American town of Roseto, Pennsylvania, which we described in chapter 3. Roseto attracted the attention of epidemiologists in the 1960s because its health was much better than that of neighboring towns (Bruhn and Wolf 1979). In particular, Rosetans had a much lower death rate from heart disease, which could not be explained by differences in smoking or diet. After a major investigation, the researchers concluded that the explanation must lie in the remarkably cohesive nature of the community—a quality they had become increasingly aware of during their work there. They said:

> From the beginning the sense of common purpose and the camaraderie among the Italians precluded ostentation or embarrassment to the less affluent, and the concern for neighbors ensured that no one was ever abandoned. This pattern of

remarkable social cohesion, in which the family as the hub and bulwark of life, provided a kind of security and insurance against catastrophe, was associated with the striking absence of myocardial infarction and sudden death. (Bruhn and Wolf 1979: 136)

In this example, an egalitarian social ethos, rather than actual equality, may also have made a contribution. At several points Bruhn and Wolf make it clear that some families were more prosperous than others but that these inequalities were not allowed to show:

During the first five years of our study it was difficult to distinguish, on the basis of dress or behavior, the wealthy from the impecunious in Roseto. Living arrangements (houses and cars) were simple and strikingly similar. Despite the affluence of many, there was no atmosphere of "keeping up with the Joneses" in Roseto. (82)

A little further on they say:

[W]e were aware that many in Roseto, mainly blouse mill owners, were relatively affluent, but . . . we were not able to identify them from their dress, speech, or manner. Nor did their houses betray evidence of affluence. . . . There appeared to be an unspoken social taboo against any display of wealth. (110)

So here, although there were significant differences in affluence, it was regarded as unseemly for the better-off to display their greater wealth and make those less well-off feel at a disadvantage.

> Proper behavior by those Rosetans who have achieved material wealth or occupational prestige requires attention to a delicate balance between ostentation and reserve, ambition and restraint, modesty and dignity. . . . The local priest emphasized that when preoccupation with earning money exceeded the unmarked boundary it became a basis for social rejection, irrespective of the standing of the person outside the community. Similarly, a lack of concern for community needs, especially by those who would spend their money on frivolous pleasures, constituted grounds for social exclusion. Rosetan culture thus provided a set of checks and balances to ensure that neither success nor failure got out of hand. (79–80)

One of the interesting things about these remarkably insightful passages is that they show that people were perfectly aware that material differences cause embarrassment and put people at a disadvantage. There is a clear recognition that material differences become the foundations of social divisions. And it is particularly interesting that here it is the rich rather than the poor who risked social rejection and exclusion if they behaved immodestly and flaunted their affluence.

Roseto appears to have been an example of a society held together not so much by actual equality, but by an egalitarian social ethos that avoided putting the less well-off at a disadvantage. But while that seems to have been true during the period of the epidemiological investigation, it seems likely that the egalitarian values would have been under strain as soon as more substantial income inequalities developed in the community. In such a situation you would wonder how long the social values could hold out against the material differences: if they were at loggerheads, which would win out? The answer soon became apparent: the cohesive social values seem to have been the legacy of the first generation of Rosetans who arrived, with few resources, from Roseto in southern Italy in the 1880s. Interestingly, they came from a part of Italy that Banfield (1958) had characterized as very uncohesive, but in their new circumstances, linguistically isolated from the rest of American society, they were thrown back on mutual support. However, as later generations of young people came to speak English as their first language and were increasingly integrated into the wider American society, they adopted its values and presumably measured themselves in relation to it. A later study showed that by the late 1980s, both the health advantage and the cohesive values apparent in the late 1960s had disappeared (Egolf et al. 1992).

In chapter 2 we saw that Tocqueville, describing his visit to the United States in 1831, had no doubt that the strength of civic community life that so impressed him was based on what he called "the equality of conditions" (see p. 37). There is no doubt that he saw the material similarities or differences as causal. He thought people in different social classes lived too differently from each other to identify with each other's feelings. People who could immediately put themselves in the shoes of others in their own class would be much less likely to do so across a material and class divide. The processes involved look much like the powerful psychological tendencies that lead to the formation of in-groups and out-groups (Tajfel et al. 1971). The social dominance processes behind social stratification clearly link up with this group psychology. Indeed, much of the psychology of group identification processes also leads us to see ourselves as members of superior or inferior groups.

We can now see how inequality, class, and the way we

know ourselves through each other's eyes (chapter 3) come together. Because we experience ourselves socially through each other's eyes, inequality goes to the heart of our sociality. Rather than being distant, external and impersonal, issues of social status and inequality are joined seamlessly to the way we are socially—and most personally—constituted. The world is not conveniently divided into an impersonal public sphere and an intimate personal one, as so much psychological and psychoanalytic theory seems to assume it is: both have an overwhelmingly personal impact. Among our prehuman ancestors there was no division between public and private spheres: the dominance hierarchy was a hierarchy of personal, face-to-face dominance and subordination.

As money becomes the sole arbiter of status, inferiority and superiority are increasingly defined through the market and what we have to spend. Money enables people to buy a sense of superiority, and it is remarkable how much the experience of luxury, whether in restaurants, in hotels, or on vacation, is advertised in terms of social exclusivity and designed to appeal to the desire to be made to feel special and to be treated as highly esteemed and valued. You buy a sense of superiority for an evening, for a few days away on vacation or, as Frank (1999) so capably explains, through possession of luxury goods. The fault is not, of course, in our desire to be valued by others. Rather, it is in the commercial exploitation, within a framework of ranking and inequality, of the unsatisfied need to be valued, which should be satisfied through genuinely social processes among equals.

7

Gender, Race, and Inequality
Kicking Down

So far we have discussed the effects of inequality almost wholly in terms of how it impacts society as a whole and those nearer the bottom of the hierarchy. But how does it affect other sections of the population? What effect does it have on ethnic minorities? How does it affect the position of women? And what does it do to men?

Some of the answers are surprising. Although more unequal societies are more male-dominated and the position of women deteriorates relative to men, men's death rates are even more adversely affected by inequality than women's. Similarly, it is also almost certainly true that social relations among men are more damaged by inequality than social relations among women. In other words, it looks as if men are harmed even more by male domination than women are. That is because inequality increases status competition among men. Not only is it a small minority of men who gain the advantages of high status, but increased status competition has a profound effect on the development and expression of masculinity: it increases the pressure on men to be tough or "hard," both physically and emotionally.

Less surprising in the fact that the health of most ethnic

minorities shows the heavy burden of their social and economic disadvantage. Ethnicity becomes a mark of a collective
social status, and its inescapability inevitably increases its
health impact. Most of the processes of racism and stigmatization are likely to increase with increasing inequality.

Gender

Let us start with the way inequality affects gender relations. It
has long been recognized that health is better where the status
of women is better (Caldwell 1986; Caldwell and Caldwell
1993; Williamson and Boehmer 1997). The most commonly
used indicator of women's status in such studies (most of
them in developing countries) was the difference between
men's and women's educational standards. What initially
seemed the most plausible explanation of how improved status for women might benefit health was that better-educated
women were likely to achieve higher standards of hygiene
and nutrition, thus lowering infant mortality rates. However,
it became clear that it was not just infant mortality that was
lower where women's status was higher. Women's death rates
were also lower.

The next hypothesis was that where women were less discriminated against, we might expect their health to be better.
But rather than improvements in the position of women
merely shifting the balance of advantage—and health—from
men to women in a kind of zero-sum game, it soon became
clear that improvements in the status of women benefited
men's health just as much as women's. Using international
cross-sectional data, Williamson and Boehmer (1997) found
that women's status explained almost as much of the differ-

ences in life expectancy among men as among women. In societies where women's status was closer to men's, both men and women had better health. The same picture has also emerged from an analysis of the data for the fifty U.S. states. Kawachi and others (1999) used three measures of women's status: proportion of elected representatives who are female, male/female pay differentials, and an index of economic autonomy. They found that the states in which women's status was good on any of these measures were also the states in which male death rates were low. Surprisingly, as table 7.1 shows, the status of women was even more closely related to men's than to women's death rates.

Table 7.1
Relation between measures of women's status and female and male mortality rates in the fifty U.S. states

Correlation coefficients		
Measures of women's status	Female mortality rates	Male mortality rates
Political participation index	−0.51	−0.64
Employment and earnings index	−0.25	−0.42
Economic autonomy index	−0.42	−0.60
(All coefficients are statistically significant.)		

Source: Kawachi et al. 1999.

As Kawachi and colleagues (1999) pointed out, discussions of subordination of women by men usually focus on the disadvantages to women and the benefits to men. But if men do benefit from controlling women's labor, not doing their share of housework and child rearing, or their use of economic and political power, why is it that male mortality rates improve rather than deteriorate where women's status is higher? Why does men's health benefit when they lose some of these apparent advantages?

The key to understanding the gender dimension of this is that women's status suffers where there is a stronger dominance hierarchy among men. Where there is a stronger dominance hierarchy among men, women will also be more dominated. In a more aggressive culture, where male power is what counts, women will be more subordinated and have lower status relative to men. Only in more egalitarian and sociable societies, where physical power, position, and authority count for less, does women's status have any real chance of improving. Advances in women's status depend on reducing competition for dominance between men.

Why men's health improves even more than women's where the status of women is better is because dominance hierarchies are power competitions among men. Men do more of the fighting and striving for dominance and suffer more of the injuries, anxieties, and stresses of these social processes. The costs are shown in their increased levels of violence, more risk-taking behavior (from car crashes to sexually transmitted diseases), excessive drinking, drug taking, and cardiovascular diseases. Because men are the rivals in the struggle for dominance, the nature of masculinity itself is deeply affected by the amount of inequality.

Accordingly, women's status suffers where there is more inequality among men not simply because they lose out physically and economically. Women also suffer because men who feel subordinated will often try to regain a sense of their authority by subordinating women, particularly their partners. This is part of a much wider process of downward discrimination in which people who feel humiliated try to repair their sense of selfhood by demonstrating their superiority over any more vulnerable group, whether women, ethnic minorities, or low-status minorities.

Most of the evidence behind this interpretation has to do with the indications that more unequal societies have a more aggressively male culture, which shows up particularly in masculine causes of death. We have seen (in chapter 2) that social relations in more egalitarian societies tend to be less hostile and more hospitable. In addition, the causes of death most closely related to income inequality include deaths from violence, accidents, and alcohol (Kaplan et al. 1996; McIsaac et al. 1997; Walberg et al. 1998; Wilkinson 1996b). Raised mortality from causes such as these is likely to affect men more than women, and probably young single men most of all. This is likely to be why alcohol and violence stood out as the fastest-growing causes of death in Eastern Europe during the 1970s and 1980s, and also why the rise in death rates was concentrated among single people and particularly single men (Watson 1996; Hajdu et al. 1995; Wilkinson 1996b).

Accidents, violence, and alcohol-related deaths such as cirrhosis reflect what we might regard as a particularly "male" culture. I have argued elsewhere (Wilkinson 1999) that there is a "culture of inequality" that is not only more violent and aggressive, but also more macho. More unequal societies are tougher, more competitive, dog-eat-dog societies. A graph in Putnam's *Bowling Alone* shows that in U.S. states with lower levels of social capital (the more unequal areas), a higher proportion of men think they would "do better than average in a fist fight." As Putnam (2000) points out, places with low social capital are more pugnacious. Imagine the difference (shown in figure 2.1) between what social relations feel like in more egalitarian societies, where only 10 percent of the population say they cannot trust others, and in the less egalitarian ones, where 35 or 40 percent say they cannot trust others (Kawachi et al. 1997).

In the past, these same tough, aggressive, macho societies were often the societies in which family honor was paramount, and men's domination of women was inextricably bound up with the male need to protect the "honor" of the women in their family by "chaperoning" them or limiting their freedom, primarily against the incursions of other men. So-called honor killings have often been part of societies in which family honor leads to feuding, vendettas, and the sacrifice of "dishonored" women.

Long before Putnam's study of social capital in Italy (Putnam, Leonardi, and Nanetti 1993), Banfield (1958) studied peasant culture in a part of southern Italy that Putnam later showed had particularly low social capital. Banfield characterized the culture as one of "amoral familism," where intense clanlike family loyalties and nepotism took precedence over any moral duty owed to the wider society. The same phrase, "amoral familism," was also used to describe how the culture was changing in Poland during the 1970s and 1980s as civil society declined and social life become increasingly private (Tarkowska and Tarkowski 1991). In general, the empirical evidence suggests that rather than being built on strong family relations, on the so-called strong ties of family, wider social capital is built on the decline of the family and the strengthening of the "weak ties" of other social relationships and moralities.

Whether more unequal societies are clannish, as they tended to be at earlier stages in economic development, or whether they come closer to the kind of social breakdown found in the concrete jungle of modern urban societies, it is easy to see why they are unlikely to lead to improvements in the status of women. Where competition between men is intensified, women lose out. A public sphere that is more aggressive and less sociable, that places a higher premium on male attributes (whether used in defense or attack), and in which women feel unable to walk around without risk of being preyed on is obviously not the kind of social environment likely to be conducive to improvements in the status of women.

These patterns show up clearly in the statistics. The paper (Kawachi et al. 1999) from which table 7.1 is taken also showed that women's status tended to be highest in the U.S. states where income inequalities were smaller. Similarly, in a group of eight developed countries, Blau and Kahn (1992) found evidence of similar relationships internationally: the bigger the overall income inequalities in a country, the more women's pay lags behind men's. The authors concluded that American women suffer a larger pay disadvantage than women in a number of other developed counties because the United States has such large income inequalities across society as a whole.

In an unpublished analysis designed to test this interpretation, Bruce Kennedy and I used official data for the fifty U.S. states and found that the amount of income inequality in each state made even more difference to men's death rates than women's. For any given decline in inequality, men's death rates fell twice as much as women's. The causes of death that contributed most to the narrowing of sex difference in life expectancy in states with more unequal incomes were lung cancer, infections (including hepatitis, AIDS, and tuberculosis), homicide, chronic liver disease and cirrhosis, and automobile accidents. This is much the same mix that other studies have reported as particularly sensitive to inequality, despite using data from very different settings (Kennedy, Kawachi, and Brainerd 1998; McIsaac et al. 1997; Walberg et al. 1998; Wilkinson 1996a).

Using data for thirty-seven countries of Eastern and Western Europe, Bobak and Marmot (1996) found that life expectancy in these countries was related to the size of the sex difference in death rates and to income inequality. They found that where life expectancy was longer, men's mortality disadvantage (and consequently the male-female mortality gap) was smaller (r = −0.72). During the 1970s and 1980s, when death rates either rose or failed to improve in Eastern Europe, there was (as we saw in the last chapter) a marked deterioration in standards of public life and civic society (Wilkinson 1996a).

The causes of excess male mortality in more unequal places speaks loudly of a more masculine culture. The picture of more smoking, drinking, road crashes, violence, risky sex, and drugs obviously contains an important element of male behavior, although none of these activities is exclusively male. We can conclude, then, that the most likely explanation of why health is better in places where women's status is higher is that women's status serves as a marker for the more egalitarian and sociable societies where not only has women's status improved, but health—particularly men's—is less affected by the costs of male competition for dominance.

What is surprising is how these processes affect even children. As many developed societies have become more unequal over the last quarter of a century or so, boys' educational performance has tended to decline relative to girls'. At one time girls did better than boys only when learning to read and write at elementary school. At older ages, and in all except the most "feminine" subjects, they were overtaken by boys. However, the balance has now shifted dramatically. Girls have been doing better than boys at older and older ages and in more and more subjects. In public exams their lead extended from the more "feminine" subjects into the gender-neutral ones and, lastly, into traditionally "male" subjects such as math and the sciences. In many of the more unequal countries, girls now maintain their lead all the way through to college. Meanwhile, more and more children—and in each case predominantly boys—are identified as having attention deficit hyperactivity disorder, disruptive behavioral problems, learning difficulties, and dyslexia, or are just plain absent. Although girls are clearly affected by the development of a very tough youth culture as well as by the special stresses of home life for the 20 percent or so of children brought up in poverty, boys are affected even more. The issue is not primarily about which sex is doing best; it is instead to point out that even in childhood the adverse effects of the more masculine culture of inequality impacts particularly on boys.

The "Bicycling Reaction"

The link we have been discussing between dominance relations among men and the status of women is part of a broader picture of the social processes by which increased inequality and dominance relations lead to more discrimination against any vulnerable group, including ethnic minorities.

Accounts of dominance behavior among nonhuman primates that form hierarchies—such as chimpanzees, macaques, and baboons—often contain descriptions of animals which, having lost a battle for status or having been attacked by a higher-ranking animal, immediately attack subordinate animals in what was usually dismissed as a display of "displaced aggression." Surprised by the frequency of these accounts, I asked Volker Sommer, a distinguished primatologist, about this. He replied:

> The phenomenon is termed *Radfahrer-Reaktion* in German (bicycling reaction), because animals show their backs to the top while kicking towards the bottom. It is very common in nonhuman primates that they, after having received aggression from a higher ranking individual, will redirect aggression towards lower ranking ones. It can be a real chain reaction: alpha slaps beta, beta slaps gamma, gamma slaps delta, delta slaps the observer! (personal communication, 1997)

The image is based, of course, on someone leaning forward on a racing bike, as if bowing to superiors, while kicking down on inferiors. But it was not until several years later that I realized that the term "bicycling reaction" originally came not from animal studies but from Adorno's *The Authoritarian*

Personality, which was an attempt to understand the workings of Nazi society and the scapegoating of the Jews in the Holocaust.

There is a widespread tendency for those who have been most humiliated, who have had their sense of selfhood most reduced by low social status, to try to regain it by asserting their superiority over any weaker or more vulnerable groups. From that point of view it works like snobbery or any other expression of downward prejudice through which people try to retain or gain status. Your status is just as much a matter of whom you place yourself above as it is of whom you find yourself below, and asserting your superiority over others is an attempt to enhance your own status. Signs of the recognition of these processes in everyday life are common. It is encapsulated in the saying "The captain kicks the cabin boy, and the cabin boy kicks the cat." We talk about people having to "take it out on someone else," and we know that bullies at school have often been given a hard time and put down by others at home or elsewhere. Among the wild baboons he studies, Sapolsky says that "such third-party displaced aggression accounts for a huge percentage of baboon violence. A middle ranking male gets trounced in a fight, turns and chases a subadult male, who lunges at an adult female, who bites a juvenile, who slaps an infant" (1998: 291).

Human examples of the bicycling reaction include the tendency for racial discrimination and racist attacks to be most frequent in times of high unemployment and economic hardship—when more people feel their dignity and status is threatened by relative poverty. In the United States, racial prejudice has been shown to be worst in the states where income differences are greatest (Kennedy et al. 1997). But per-

haps where this "bicycling reaction" is most clearly demonstrated is in prisons. Prisoners are among the most shamed
and humiliated groups in society, and there are few people
over whom they can assert superiority and regain some sense
of themselves. This often leads to strong dominance competition and violence in prisons, but the group over whom most
prisoners feel they can assert their supremacy is sex offenders.
As a result, sex offenders often have to be housed separately to
protect them from attacks from other prisoners. It is as if people are saying, "At least I'm better than those bastards."

There are many accounts in feminist literature of how humiliated men are more likely to use violence against women.
The following example comes from the borders of Mexico
and New Mexico, where the term *macho* originated. Gloria
Anzaldúa wrote:

> For men like my father, being "macho" meant being strong
> enough to protect and support my mother and us, yet being
> able to show love. Today's macho has doubts about his ability
> to feed and protect his family. His "machismo" is an adapta-
> tion to oppression and poverty and low self-esteem. It is the
> result of hierarchical male dominance. The Anglo, feeling in-
> adequate and inferior and powerless, displaces or transfers
> these feelings to the Chicano by shaming him. In the Gringo
> world, the Chicano suffers from excessive humility and self-
> effacement, shame of self and self-deprecation.
>
> The loss of a sense of dignity and respect in the macho
> breeds a false machismo which leads him to put down
> women and even to brutalize them. Coexisting with his sex-
> ist behavior is a love of the mother which takes precedence
> over that of all others. Devoted son, macho pig. To wash
> down the shame of his acts, of his very being, and to handle

the brute in the mirror, he takes to the bottle, the snort, the needle and the fist. (1987: 83)

The other side of this coin is, of course, that risks of domestic violence are lower in more egalitarian and cohesive societies. As well as showing that domestic violence was associated with more patriarchal attitudes, Dobash and colleagues (1992) showed that the risk of violence was lower where such attitudes were weaker, and that more egalitarian partnerships have a lower risk of violence. Finkler (1997) found that domestic conflict was associated not only with alcohol consumption but also with lack of community sanctions and men's inferior social status (in relation to other men). On all three counts we would expect this to mean that inequality would increase rates of domestic violence: alcohol consumption increases in response to the social breakdown resulting from greater inequality, inequality decreases involvement in community life, and inequality also increases the burden of low social status for those at the bottom. Hence Levinson (1989), who looked at sixteen small-scale, preindustrial, non-patriarchal societies, found that there were virtually no reports of domestic violence among them. Finally, although between 10 and 20 percent of couples in the United States reported domestic violence sometime during their marriage, victimization rates were found to be twice as high among women married to men employed in highly hierarchical and authoritarian settings such as the armed forces (Brannen et al. 1999).

It looks as if dominance works in much the same way whether we look at relations between individuals or those between groups. As Sidanius and Pratto (1999) said, it is a universal grammar of social power and accounts for "the major forms of intergroup conflict, such as racism, classism and patriarchy."

Race

Socioeconomic inequalities often lead to differences in ethnicity, race, religion, or language, which might otherwise be easily accepted, becoming infected with social prejudice. However, where material inequalities are smaller, issues of social superiority and inferiority are less in the foreground of social relations and religious, ethnic, racial, and linguistic differences are less likely to cause friction.

The power of status differences to stigmatize what would otherwise seem unimportant physical or cultural differences has been demonstrated a number of times—most famously by Jane Elliot (1996) in a classroom experiment in the 1960s. She deliberately established a superiority/inferiority distinction between "superior" brown-eyed and "inferior" blue-eyed children and found that within half an hour the confidence, demeanor, and performance of children was affected according to which group they were in.

In the United States the African American population has suffered the brunt of economic inequalities that are larger there than in any other developed country. Partly as a result, average life expectancy in the richest white areas is sixteen years longer than in the poorest black areas (Geronimus et al. 2001). The poorest black areas have death rates higher at most ages than in rural Bangladesh (McCord et al. 1990). Official figures show a difference in average life expectancy between the black and white populations of the United States of be-

tween five and six years. When controlling statistically for income and/or education, the standard epidemiological studies
usually find that social status explains most, but not quite all,
of blacks' disadvantage in life expectancy. Race is not, however, a genetically meaningful category in the United States.
All human beings are genetically 99.9 percent the same, and
each of us has more in common genetically with some people
who have a different skin color than we do with some who
have the same. Skin color reflects the power of the social
meanings attached to it. In many societies a similar burden of
class prejudice has become attached to more ephemeral and
less conspicuous differences such as accent and other aspects
of appearance that have been stigmatized. The important difference is that although people can, to varying degrees,
change many of the cultural markers of class when they move
up socially, skin color is indelible. This is why African Americans who live in predominantly white areas, where they are
likely to feel both more conspicuous and more discriminated
against, tend to have less good health even though they are
better off. This so-called group density effect—which we discussed in chapter 6—is hard to explain except in terms of the
extent to which people do or don't feel at ease and accepted
in their social environment.

Income differences and skin color clearly interact in the
social processes of stigmatization, prejudice, and discrimination. Bigger income differences increase the stigmatization of
skin color. This is why there is more racial prejudice (and
worse health for blacks and whites) in American states where
income differences are larger. In a study by Kennedy and colleagues (1997) prejudice was measured using questions from
the General Social Survey that asked people what they

thought were the reasons why, "on the average, blacks have worse income, jobs and housing than white people." The explanations people in the more unequal states were more likely to choose were very like the attitudes that produce high scores on the Social Dominance Orientation Scale (Sidanius and Pratto 1999). People who are more racially prejudiced, such as those who score high on the Social Dominance Orientation Scale, are more likely to believe that people's social position reflects their innate abilities or inabilities rather than different life chances, discrimination, or injustice. Where material differences are greater, processes of social distancing and differentiation are stronger and all characteristics associated with low social status, including skin color, become more stigmatized.

Income inequality in U.S. states and cities is strongly associated with worse health among whites as well as blacks. That is to say that everyone's health—black and white—is worse where there is more income inequality. Life is more affected by social divisions and social hierarchy, and not just between ethnic groups. Where there is more income inequality in the population as a whole, there is also (as you would expect) a bigger difference between average black and white incomes. Where a higher proportion of the population is black, income differences tend to be bigger, and some have pointed out that health in the United States is, on some statistical bases, even more closely related to the proportion of the population which is black than to income inequality (Deaton and Lubotsky 2003). The problem, of course, is not ethnicity but the social prejudices that take place around it. Given the history of racism, sometimes the proportion of the population that is black may tell us even more than income differentials about how big a problem there is of status differentials in a society. The data imply that the feedback effects between racism and inequality are more powerful where the black population forms a larger minority.

Kerala

A society that perhaps shows most clearly how smaller income inequalities can reduce tension across religious, caste, and ethnic divisions is the Indian state of Kerala, on the west coast, near the tip of the Indian subcontinent. With a population of about thirty-two million, Kerala has long been known as India's most egalitarian state. It elected communist governments for four periods in the second half of the twentieth century, and as a coastal state, it had many fishing cooperatives. Now cooperatives make up a substantial part of every sector of the economy. The state has undergone extensive land redistribution programs, abolishing landlordism and redistributing land to peasants; it subsidizes rice for the poor; it has a high minimum wage, and—partly as a result of a massive literacy campaign started in 1989 with more than 350,000 volunteers—it has achieved over 90 percent literacy levels. Kerala is also matriarchal, and the status of women, on many different measures, is higher than in any other Indian state. High levels of literacy are thought to have increased women's participation in public life. Both Kerala's relative equality and the high status of its women have long histories. Despite levels of income that until recently were lower than the Indian average (but have recently caught up), it has outstandingly good levels of life expectancy. With a GNP of scarcely $1,000 per person per year, in the late 1990s life expectancy for men and women in Kerala was nonetheless only three or four years less than in the United States. Japanese life expectancy exceeded that in the United States by a greater margin.

As well as good health and smaller income differences, Kerala has many of the characteristics associated with high social capital, including high status for women. It has the highest consumption of newspapers per head of population in India (one of the measures of social capital used by Putnam in his Italian study), and what Ashutosh Varshney described as "a remarkable civicness, a great associational life." Varshney likened Kerala to the America observed by Tocqueville in the nineteenth century. He described it as a society filled with "associations . . . of a thousand kinds, religious, moral, serious, futile, general or restricted, enormous or diminutive" (Kapur 1998: 44). It has soccer clubs, film clubs, youth clubs, tea shops, public libraries in every village, political associations, and activist groups, some with membership running into thousands; membership is almost a civic obligation. In addition, more progress has been made in Kerala in overcoming the scourge of "untouchability" than in any other part of India, and large Muslim, Christian, and Hindu communities have lived side by side with comparatively little strife.

If we were to doubt whether the strength of community life is really linked to the weakening of dominance relations, there is a particularly interesting indicator of it in Kerala. As well as the evidence of greater economic equality and the improved status of women, there is also evidence that people resist the subordination of class and the employer/employee relationship. You get a strong impression of people unwilling to be cowed. Writing—not always flatteringly—in the *Atlantic Monthly,* Akash Kapur (1998) said, "Kerala is a proud state, devoid of the self-abasement which often comes with poverty. Beggars are rare. Women in Kerala will look one in the eye." But then he also said, "People know their rights. . . . Shopkeepers and hotel clerks can be astoundingly rude: service is not a notion that comes easily to the Keralite laborer. . . . This refusal to serve is at the root of strikes by disgruntled workers" (44). Company directors lament the difficulties of working with "overeducated and overly assertive laborers." Despite its good economic performance, Kapur describes it as "a good place to live, but a tough place to do business" (45). Laborers in Kerala come from an ethical culture partly informed by the large number of cooperatives in the economy, whereas the employers, coming from outside Kerala, have been used to a more subservient labor force.

Kerala's mixture of pride, equality, the high status of women, and good health leaves little room to doubt that these features move together and are related to each other as we have suggested. In addition, as we shall see in chapter 9, the extent to which the presence of cooperatives can affect local values has recently been shown in a study of three towns around Bologna in northern Italy.

In this chapter we have seen how inequality can interact with other intergroup processes, affecting the attitudes to and treatment of any more vulnerable groups—whether defined by race, religion, or gender. Such differences—which as differences between equals in a nonhierarchical setting may give rise to little or no prejudice and friction—often become highly charged when overlaid with economic differences that cast relations between the groups in terms of superiority and inferiority.

We have also seen how, through the so-called bicycling reaction, these processes are exacerbated among people who, having been rendered inferior by those above them, try to regain some sense of self-worth by asserting their superiority over individuals or groups they can put down by overt violence or other discriminatory processes. In this sense, we should perhaps recognize that the processes that lead to lynchings or some of the grossest expressions of prejudice may start at the top of society with much milder forms of social exclusion and snobbishness.

8
Evolved Social Strategies
Mutuality and Dominance

Prehistoric Equality

Human beings are neither naturally egalitarian nor naturally hierarchical. Historically and prehistorically, we have lived in every kind of society, from the most authoritarian and tyrannical to the most egalitarian. But there are (as we shall see) clear evolutionary reasons why this dimension of the social environment matters to us as much as it does—why we are particularly attentive and sensitive to status differences and cannot easily ignore them.

The fact that this psychological sensitivity to status has an evolutionary basis does not mean that we are condemned to live in dominance hierarchies or that change is impossible. Quite the reverse. As well as explaining why this aspect of the quality of social relations is so important to us, it also helps us understand why we have very different responses to social environments according to the extent of equality or inequality within them. So rather than an understanding of the evolutionary roots of these patterns implying that they are fixed, it shows us instead the key to progress: what we need to change in the social structure in order to produce desirable changes in social behavior and in the quality of social relations.

Many of the early applications of evolutionary theory to human behavior were rejected by progressive opinion because they seemed to biologize existing social arrangements and give them a spurious legitimacy. By suggesting that various aspects of society were unavoidable expressions of human nature, they implied that it would be futile to attempt to change them. But evolutionary psychology is a field that, like any other, has both progressive and conservative possibilities, and the argument should not be allowed to become monopolized by just one side of the political debate.

Marx and Engels opened *The Communist Manifesto* of 1848 with the resounding sentences: "The history of all hitherto existing society is the history of class struggles. Freeman and slave, patrician and plebeian, lord and serf, guild-master and journeyman, in a word, oppressor and oppressed, stood in constant opposition to one another." However, although the history of all hitherto existing *historical* societies might be the history of class struggle, the same cannot be said of the societies of prehistory. For at least 90 percent of the time we have existed as anatomically modern human beings, with brains as large as they are now, the evidence suggests that we lived in highly egalitarian societies.

David Erdal and Andrew Whiten reviewed the evidence on equality taken from over a hundred accounts of twenty-four recent hunting and gathering societies spread over four continents. They concluded that

> egalitarian behaviour is one of the most clearly documented universals. Over 100 particular observations document the unique nature of human hunter-gatherer egalitarianism, demonstrating an absence of social hierarchy and a sharing of

resources which goes beyond the explanatory power of either kinship or reciprocation. Individuals do sometimes attempt to obtain a disproportionate share of resources or influence for themselves, but this is contained through vigilance and counter-dominant behaviour by their group members.

These societies were characterized by "[e]galitarianism, cooperation and sharing on a scale unprecedented in primate evolution" (Erdal and Whiten 1996: 140). "They share food, not simply with kin or even just with those who reciprocate, but according to need even when food is scarce" (142).

> There is no dominance hierarchy among hunter-gatherers. No individuals has priority of access to food which . . . is shared. In spite of the marginal female preference for the more successful hunters as lovers, access to sexual partners is not a right which correlates with rank. In fact rank is simply not discernible among hunter-gatherers. This is a cross cultural universal, which rings out unmistakably from the ethnographic literature, sometimes in the strongest terms. (144)

Christopher Boehm had come to similar conclusions in an earlier review of the literature (Boehm 1993), and other anthropologists have called these societies "assertively egalitarian" (Woodburn 1982). Indeed, the debate among anthropologists is less about how egalitarian these societies were than it is about why later human societies became less egalitarian during the development of settled agriculture.

In attempts to fault the general thesis of equality in preagricultural societies, some commentators, often from outside the field, have pointed to particular foraging societies where there are signs of small status differences, where some people

are listened to more than others, or where there are some cer-
emonial goods that confer status. Others have suggested that
at such low levels of economic development societies had few
possessions that could be distributed unequally, and still others have suggested that the typical group size was too small for
there to be enough people for substantial inequalities to
emerge. But none of these arguments recognizes the fact that
there are a great many animal species—including many nonhuman primates—that establish very strict dominance hierarchies, despite living in small groups and having nothing but
food and sexual partners to be unequal with. Among them it
is normal practice for weaker animals to have to wait—however hungry—until dominant animals have had their fill of
whatever food may be available. It is also common for dominant males to herd the females and drive off weaker males to
exclude them from mating. Not giving way to a dominant
animal in either situation results in a vicious attack. In contrast, there is absolutely no suggestion anywhere in the literature that social systems in any human foraging societies
worked even remotely like this. Instead, there is complete
agreement on the ubiquity of systems of food sharing and gift
exchange, relationships of mutuality that reflect social relations based on totally different principles. Not only that, but
neither is there any suggestion that, among hunter-gatherers,
high-status men had harems, or that the poor were left to
starve while the rich had more than enough, although both
are common enough in later forms of society. Indeed, in most
foraging societies the extent of food sharing and gift exchange makes it impossible to talk about distinct groups of
rich and poor in the same societies. Not only was there a high
degree of equality, but social relations were not overt power

relations ordered according to the ability to be physically threatening—either in the way that animal pecking orders are, or as many of the more tyrannical dominance hierarchies in preindustrial societies were. Instead they were based on patterns of indebtedness and social obligation.

But despite so much evidence of egalitarianism and few, if any, indications of more than marginal differences in power, possessions, or sexual access (none of which arose from the systematic use of physical threats), many people now find it hard to believe this picture of human prehistory. Why some find it so hard to accept is often because they make the mistaken assumption that an egalitarian society, based on food sharing and gift exchange, could only have existed on the basis of an implausibly altruistic human nature—quite unlike the acquisitive self-interestedness we see in modern societies. But that is a misunderstanding of the basis of this equality: it is rather as if people in foraging societies were to believe that the inequality in modern societies must reflect either a remarkable altruism among the poorest half of the population or continuous repressive violence. Why else, they might ask, would the poorest half of the population put up with getting just 20 percent of society's income while the richest half gets the remaining 80 percent?

What has changed since the beginning of agriculture is not human nature, but the environment within which it operates. Rather than being based on altruism, sharing in foraging societies is said to have been "vigilant" sharing (people watching to see that they get their fair share). And equality was maintained similarly, through what has been described as a "counterdominance" strategy through which people protected their autonomy.

Christopher Boehm (1993, 1999) went through a vast body of anthropological literature, covering not only foraging societies but also the less completely egalitarian early agricultural societies, in order to see how these societies maintained their equality. He looked for accounts of what happened when someone did take on a rather overbearing, bossy, or leadership role. What he found was that such people were teased, ridiculed, ostracized, physically attacked, or even killed. He concluded that these societies used a "counterdominance" strategy: the whole society acted as an alliance of everyone against anyone who started to take on a dominant role. It was as if the strategy that sometimes leads to two or three monkeys forming an alliance to depose the dominant male had been generalized across the whole society, so that it functioned as an alliance of everyone against anyone who took on a dominant role.

Boehm suggested that what motivated people to use a counterdominance strategy was a desire to maintain their autonomy, which is fiercely guarded among foragers. Gardner said a strong emphasis on individual autonomy characterized "Holocene hunters, fishers, and gatherers in general, and the extreme emphasis on it which is reported for certain foragers in Asia, Africa, and North America" (1991: 543). He also described what he called the "rank concession syndrome" that occurs when a whole society which had remained isolated and intact suddenly loses its autonomy and is turned into an appendage of a wider, more advanced society. He described how the process "entails accepting social inferiority and relative powerlessness, adopting practices of the dominant . . . and losing solidarity in the process" (546).

Not only is autonomy closely related to equity in that a

precondition for autonomy is the need to avoid subservience and subordination, but it also comes up in research literature from a number of different fields emphasizing the importance of a sense of control. As we saw in chapter 3, studies of health at work have shown that not having control over one's work is damaging to health (Marmot et al. 1997; Karasek et al. 1990; Stam et al. 2002–2003; Bobak et al. 1998). Having a sense of control is more about social than natural limitations on one's freedom: what matters is not being under someone's thumb. The protest—particularly common from children—of "Don't tell me what to do" is surely a protest against an infringement of one's autonomy.

After discussing how much confidence could be placed in attempts to infer from the social organization of recent hunter-gatherers to prehistoric ones, Erdal and Whiten produced an illustrative graph of the human transition from dominance hierarchies to equality during some unspecified period of early human prehistory, and then from equality back to dominance hierarchies during the course of agricultural development. While there can be no doubt about the rough timing of the ending of egalitarianism and the emergence of class societies since the development of agriculture, there is very little evidence as to when, in our prehistory, human beings first became egalitarian. There are nonetheless a few clues.

Skeletal remains suggest that around two or three million years ago our male ancestors were about 30 percent taller than our female ancestors. During the next million years this height differential reduced to 8 percent (Relethford 2003). In many animal species a larger size differential between males and females reflects the existence of dominance hierarchies in which reproductive access to females is monopolized by larger dominant males: because dominant males tend to be larger than others and to have a reproductive advantage, males in species that have dominance hierarchies tend to get progressively larger than females. If the prehistoric reduction in the sex difference in height among our ancestors indicates that dominant males no longer monopolized a disproportionate share of the breeding, it suggests that more egalitarian social systems may have emerged around two million years ago.

Another factor that perhaps points in the same direction is the growth of the human brain and our growing dependency on learning and culture. Not only did the increasing size of the human skull determine the length of time a baby could grow before being born, but a greater reliance on learning meant a longer period of child dependency. This in turn would have increased women's need for more paternal investment in child rearing and weighed against mating with a dominant male in favor of pair bonding. The development of pair bonding is almost certainly linked to changes in female sexuality: to the development of hidden ovulation, almost continuous sexual receptivity of human females, and perhaps also the tendency for ovulation to synchronize among women living together. In an important sense all these changes were part of the development of a nonhierarchical biology, a more egalitarian sexuality, which made it harder for dominant males to monopolize the reproductive potential of a significant number of females. Although a dominant male can fight—with some success—to control access to females during a brief sexually receptive and obvious estrus, the odds would be heavily against him if the time of ovulation was unknown and females were sexually receptive all the time.

Pair bonding must have been part of the move away from male dominance systems toward the development of egalitarianism, and it was almost certainly mediated by changes in female sexuality which made it harder for dominant males to monopolize females. As well as being a response to the growth of the human brain, pair bonding enabled further postnatal growth of the brain and some of the results of that also favored equality. For example, the development of tools, particularly primitive weapons, would have had a strongly democratic effect. Weapons and greater intelligence made differences in physical size much less important. Even simple weapons such as clubs, spears, or axes enable anyone, weak or strong, to come up to people unawares, perhaps in their sleep, and kill them with a single blow. With weapons, the muscular strength and size that had been the mark of the dominant male could no longer guarantee safety and ensure preeminence. Instead they made everyone vulnerable to everyone else, making it necessary to conduct social relations in light of that fact.

Scarcity and the Decline of Equality in Agricultural Societies

As well as doubt about the factors that may have led to the emergence of egalitarianism in human prehistory, there is also controversy about what might have led to its decline in agricultural societies. James Woodburn's (1982) suggestion that the main practical difference between more and less egalitarian societies was whether their economy was what he called an "immediate return" or a "delayed return" system is the most influential. The distinction is between the delayed return to labor in agriculture, where you plant and look after the crop for months before you get any food from it, and the immediate return enjoyed by hunters and gatherers, who usually bring back food on the same day as they go out to get it. As well as the heavy prior investment of labor needed in agriculture, delayed return systems involve food storage and often need more tools and equipment—which again involve a prior outlay of labor to make them.

Delayed return systems clearly provide additional opportunities for private ownership of resources such as stored foods and sown fields. But the most fundamental rationale for inequality is always scarcity. Ranking systems among animals and humans alike are systems by which the strong gain prior access to resources, and the only point of competing for access to resources is the threat of scarcity. You do not need to compete for resources that are freely available and abundant, but the delayed return of agricultural systems always implies a potential for scarcity: when needs cannot be met immediately and people rely on stored food, shortages can—and often do—occur between planting and harvest.

Although it is often assumed that the development of agriculture reduced scarcity, agricultural societies are actually more prone to scarcity than foraging societies. Typically hunters and gatherers recognize a very large number of species of animals and plants as edible but normally eat only a small number of preferred species. This means that they have a lot to fall back on if any particular food species has a bad year and is in short supply. In less good times they need only eat a slightly higher proportion of species a little lower on their preference list. In contrast, not only are agricultural systems dependent on a very small range of cultivated crops, but the amount you grow reflects your guesses about the chances of a poor harvest. To be safe from occasional famine you have to grow much more than is normally necessary year after year. The prudent pattern for a subsistence farmer is to do substantially more work each year to produce crops that will, if all goes well, go to waste. But whether you grow 10 percent or 100 percent more than you usually need, there is always at least a possibility of bad harvests and crop failure with little to fall back on. And the heavier the work, the smaller the safety margin people are likely to provide for themselves. As a result, agricultural societies are much more susceptible to occasional famines than hunters and gatherers are.

People in hunting and gathering societies are now recognized as having lived well, so much so that they have been described as "the original affluent societies" (Sahlins 1974). Studies suggest that they typically had to work substantially less to feed themselves than people in agricultural societies. Rather than taking up agriculture as if it were the discovery of a superior way of life, hunters and gatherers have always known how to grow things. However, until population densities rose above the very low levels which could be sustained by hunting and gathering what grew naturally, they were able to avoid the extra work entailed in growing food crops (Boserup 1965; Wilkinson 1973; Cohen 1977). Agriculture was a response to rising population densities. The biblical story of Adam and Eve being cast out of the Garden of Eden is a mythological version of the beginnings of agriculture. In the Garden of Eden, Adam and Eve were foragers: they could "freely eat of every tree" without having to till the ground. When they were cast out, they were condemned to "till the ground" and "eat bread" in sorrow (Genesis, chapter 3) because they had broken a sexual taboo—perhaps a reference to the social constraints on reproduction which had previously kept population densities low (Wilkinson 1973). In the context of the departure from egalitarianism and the social values which went with it, the biblical concept of the Fall as a moral fall is interesting.

Mark Cohen (1977) suggests that the beginnings of agriculture were accompanied by food shortage. He points to widespread evidence of a prehistoric food crisis. His argument has received more recent support from archaeological analysis of teeth and bones showing that early agriculture was accompanied by worse health and decreased stature (Larsen 1995). Archaeological research has found evidence of health inequalities within societies indicative of important nutritional differences only since the advent of agriculture (Danforth 1999). The emergence of health inequalities reflecting differences in nutrition not only shows that these societies—unlike their predecessors—were unequal, but also confirms that the inequalities were related to sufficiently large differences in access to basic necessities to affect life chances; in other words, under agriculture, scarcity was a powerful enough force to have a real impact on the social structure.

Rather than helping us escape from the scarcity underpinning inequality, it is truer to say that most of the long history of agricultural development and the early stages of industrialization were driven by scarcity. At each stage growing population pressure forced increasingly intensive methods of exploiting the land and all land-based resources (Boserup 1965; Wilkinson 1973). Only as population densities increased further did it become necessary to keep land in continuous cultivation and to maintain soil fertility artificially by manuring and growing rotation crops. The main productive innovations, right up to the first industrial revolution in eighteenth- and early-nineteenth-century England, are best seen as the responses of societies having to cultivate increasingly intensively and having to cope with the extra workload involved.

The Social Impact of Affluence

Only during the last few generations has economic growth begun to weaken the grip of absolute poverty on society. The health effects of the decline of absolute want show up clearly enough in the epidemiological transition discussed in chapter 1. Not only is national income per capita no longer the main determinant of longevity in the rich countries, but the so-called diseases of affluence have become the diseases of the poor in affluent societies. And the greatest reward of affluence is that social stratification—based on the threat of scarcity—has also begun to lose its grip on us.

The decline of absolute want has dramatically reduced the social disciplining power of poverty and inequality. Rather than absolute destitution, the vast majority—even of the poorest 20 percent of the population in most developed countries—have televisions, refrigerators, and many other consumer durables (chapter 3, table 3.1). This means that, although in many countries income differentials have shown no long-term decline, the social impact of the same inequalities has nevertheless declined very substantially. Yet in politically regressive periods, policies that allow the reemergence of homelessness and unemployment once again act as a disciplining force, shoring up the power of the establishment. As

Tony Benn, a veteran left-wing British politician, once pointed out, "[T]hey are put there to frighten us."

In historical perspective, the trend toward greater *social* equality seems unstoppable, spanning the abolition of slavery, the development of democracy, equality before the law, the establishment of welfare states, the outlawing of discrimination on grounds of race or religion, the moves toward equal rights for gays and lesbians, the ending of capital punishment (in most developed countries), and the sharp diminution of some of the more overt signs of class distinctions and deference. The gradual improvement in the position of women seems to have the same unstoppable historical quality to it. With women's increasing political participation and the slow movement toward equality within marriage, barbarities such as the huge harems of virtually imprisoned women belonging to high-status men in many earlier civilizations (Betzig 1986), or the sexual dominance once enshrined in feudal practices such as droit du seigneur, seem from the perspective of the affluent democracies to belong to a very distant and primitive world.

However, the lack of any substantial diminution in income differentials remains a profound obstacle to the emergence of a new postscarcity humanity. In order to understand the hold inequality continues to have over us, we must understand the role it has played in the evolution of our psychology. We have seen a little of how changing circumstances have produced ages of equality and then of social stratification in human prehistory and history. Instead of limiting us to one or another form of social organization, we have evolved to be equipped with different psychological and behavioral strategies to deal with the different kinds of social environment in which we might find ourselves. The point is to identify the main influences on social behavior in modern populations.

Affiliative and Dominance Strategies

Michael Chance has drawn attention to two contrasting forms of social organization found among nonhuman primates: "an agonistically rank-ordered form, typical of baboons and macaques, and a hedonic form, typical of the great apes" (Chance and Jolly 1970: 19). Trower and colleagues (1990) have made the same distinction between different human societies—agonistic (hierarchical) societies characterized by dominance hierarchies and more egalitarian hedonic societies based on cooperation. Chance describes them as "two antithetical types of social systems" in which we "tend to function in one of two mental modes" (1988: 1). Each one of the two modes "is, at one and the same time, a property of our minds and of the corresponding way in which we relate to those about us" (3).

Agonic social systems (typified by baboons and macaques) are "based on the persistent awareness of potential threat from dominant males" (Reynolds and Luscombe 1976: 105). Chance says that among animal species with agonic social systems,

> [i]ndividuals are always together in a group yet spread out, separate from one another, keeping their distance from the more dominant ones to whom they are constantly attentive. They are ready at an instant to avoid punishment by reacting to those threats that are dealt out from time to time down the rank order. This they do with various submissive and/or appeasing gestures, and by spatial equilibration which . . . serve

to prevent escalation of threat into agonistic conflict, yet with tension and arousal remaining at a high level. The continuous high tension, without the accompanying agonistic behaviour, is the unique characteristic of this mode (1988: 6–7).

Of the great apes, perhaps bonobos (to whom we are as closely related as we are to chimps) are the best example of the hedonic form of social organization. They have been dubbed the "egalitarian" and "gentle" apes by Frans de Waal, who says the bonobo "is best characterized as a female-centered, egalitarian primate species that substitutes sex for aggression" (Waal and Lanting 1997: 4). Bonobos use sexual and erotic contact for social purposes—to reduce anxiety, ease conflict, signal friendliness, and calm stressful situations. As Waal says, "[W]hereas in most other species, sexual behavior is a fairly distinct category, in the bonobo it has become an integral part of social relationships, and not just between males and females" (Waal 1997: 4).

While the agonic modes of behavior are appropriate for dealing with power relations, threat, and fear, hedonic behavior patterns are honed to deal with social relations based on greater equality, mutual support, and reciprocity. Among most—perhaps all—primate species, social behavior involves a combination of both patterns: dominance hierarchies may be present to varying degrees, and there are also what appear to be friendships based on mutual grooming, which, as Alison Jolly (1985: 207) pointed out, "provides the social cement of primates from lemur to chimpanzee." We also know that even among nonhuman primates grooming incurs social obligations and leads to reciprocity: an animal that has been groomed by another is more likely to come to its aid when it hears the other's distress calls.

Human beings are of course also programmed for both kinds of social interaction and tend to make sharp distinctions between dominance behavior up and down the social hierarchy and affiliative behavior between equals. Rather than each of us being fixed in one or the other mode or all of us changing randomly from one to the other, our behavior reflects our understanding of the nature of the social interaction and social environment in which we find ourselves. Yet many aspects of dominance or affiliative behavior, though they may appear carefully honed, are pursued quite unconsciously. We saw in chapter 5 how reactive we can be to imputations of low social status, being disrespected, or feeling put down and ignored. We also saw the processes of social prejudice—class and racial discrimination—that come out in relation to social inferiors. In chapter 3 we saw how responsive to friendship we are: we noted the human tendency for reciprocity, saw the way friendship is symbolized by the gift, and remarked how the gift is a sign that we do not compete for scarce resources and, when reciprocated, forms something amounting to a social contract. We know that these tendencies are universal among humans. Gifts in all societies create a sense of indebtedness and need to be reciprocated. Similarly, the "loss of face" or dishonor involved in social humiliation is always hard to bear and may trigger violence. And finally, we saw how the people we choose to socialize with, make friends with, and marry tend to be our social equals: status divisions seem to make friendship more difficult.

In the words of the psychiatrically oriented Social Systems

Institute's Web page (Chance 1998), the agonic mode in human beings

> is characterised by hierarchical, authoritarian structures. Living in an agonic environment, we are predominantly interested in protecting ourselves. We are primarily concerned with self security . . . [and] rank hierarchy, convention, and maintaining good order. . . . In this mode our concerns are predominantly self-protective and engage information-processing systems in our brains that are specifically designed to attend, recognise and respond to potential threats to our physical self, status, and social presentation.

In contrast to this defensive, "insecure and fearful" mode, hedonic situations are experienced as "carefree and creative" not only because hostility is replaced by mutual support and security, but also because "group-members form a network of social relationships and are able to communicate fearlessly and openly with each other."

These two forms of social interaction are merely the two opposite extremes of the ways in which we can conduct social relations: at one pole they are a matter of power and self-interest, and at the other a matter of social investments, trust, and reciprocity. In practice, social life involves varying mixtures of the two.

It is not difficult to see the evolutionary reasons why we might expect to have an inherent tendency to be attentive to social dominance hierarchies, our position in them, and friendship. If position in a dominance hierarchy determines access to such fundamentally important scarce resources as food and reproductive opportunities, there can be no more powerful determinants of survival and reproductive success.

Similarly, friendships and social alliances must also have been crucially important both in ensuring one's security and in the struggle for access to necessities. Allies were the key not only to mutual defense but also to gaining all the other benefits of cooperation. And until a period in human evolution is identified during which all remnants of evolved dispositions were wiped from the human slate, we must assume that some are still present today.

Clearly dominance hierarchies and friendship have had different significances for men and women. While dominant males did much more than their share of breeding, differences in fertility among females are less affected by social rank. While males had to avoid what Pinker (1997) has called the "evolutionary cul de sac" of low social status, for females low status was likely to reduce their own and their offspring's survival. Indeed, among female chimpanzees, high social status has been shown to lead to substantially better reproductive performance (Pusey, Williams, and Goodall 1997). Part of the reason social rank has such dire reproductive consequences for males is of course that when males are ranked by strength, fitness, or ability to gain access to resources, it would be odd if females did not prefer more dominant males as sexual partners. Indeed, Ng and Bond (2002) have shown that in countries where income inequalities are greater, women pay more attention to things such as the financial prospects, social status, and ambition of prospective partners. The eighteenth- and nineteenth-century novels dealing with pair bonding in the context of class show how great the preoccupation with "making a good catch" can be—even if sexual attraction and wealth may try any heroine by not always leading in exactly the same direction.

The tendency for men and women to have different responses to low social status may be related to its different reproductive significance for the sexes. Responses to relative poverty and deprivation are surprisingly sex-specific: at its simplest, young men are violent and become risk takers, while young women have teenage pregnancies and get depressed. These differences stand out unmistakably in endless data sets, and both responses are related to inequality (Pickett and Wilkinson, forthcoming); we shall see more of the logic behind them later in this chapter.

The Social Brain

Friendship and social ranking have achieved their psychological hold over us not only because they are the opposite forms of social relation, but more particularly because they are opposite ways of handling the awesome potential for conflict resulting from competition for scarce resources which exists within so many species. For human beings the stakes are particularly high because the potential benefits of cooperation among us are unusually large. When Hobbes wrote *Leviathan*, in which he identified the potential for conflict over access to scarce resources as the central political problem facing human societies, he would no doubt have been surprised that bonobos had developed such a different way of avoiding conflict arising from the same source. Waal gives a vivid description of their strategy:

> As soon as caretakers at a zoo approach bonobos with food, the males develop erections. Even before the food is thrown into the enclosure, the apes are inviting one another to sex:

males invite females, females invite males, and genito-genital (GG) rubbing among females is also common. What is all this sex about?

In all animals, attractive food strains relationships. There are two reasons to believe that sexual activity is the bonobo's answer to this circumstance. First, anything, not just food, that arouses the interest of more than one bonobo may trigger sexual contact. For example, if two bonobos approach a cardboard box given to them, they will briefly mount each other before playing with the box. I have even seen adult females GG-rub when one had only found a little piece of frayed rope and another hurried over for a closer look. Such situations often cause squabbles in other species, whereas bonobos are quite tolerant. They use sex to . . . change the tone of the encounter.

Second, sex often occurs in aggressive situations that have nothing to do with food. For example, after one male has chased another away from a female, the two may engage in a scrotal rub. Or when one female has hit a juvenile, and the juvenile's mother has come to its defence, the problem may be resolved by intense GG-rubbing between the two adults. Based on hundreds of such incidents, my study produced the first solid evidence for sexual behavior as a mechanism to overcome social tensions. This function is not absent in other animals (or humans, for that matter), but the art of sexual reconciliation may well have reached its evolutionary peak in the bonobo. (1997: 109)

This passage shows not only the potential for conflict between members of the same species who have all the same needs, but also what is clearly another evolved response to solving it. Neurological research has started to identify ways in which human brains are built to reinforce cooperative behavior. An experiment in which magnetic resonance imaging was used to scan the brains of women playing the trust game Prisoner's Dilemma found that mutual cooperation activated brain areas linked to reward processing, suggesting that neural networks positively reinforce reciprocal altruism and help motivate people to resist the temptation to accept one-sided favors without reciprocation (Rilling et al. 2002).

A dramatic illustration of the importance of getting social relations right comes from archaeological research on the growth of the human brain. The leading explanations of the evolutionary expansion of the early human brain suggest that its growth was stimulated by the demands of social life (Byrne 1995). Across a wide range of mammalian species Eisenberg (1981) showed that more social species tended to have brains which were larger in proportion to body size than those in less social species. Perhaps because all higher primates have enormous brains for their body size and are highly social (Lee 1996), it is only among them that this relationship does not hold. In its place, Dunbar (1992) has show that among primates, the larger the group size, the larger the size of the neocortex in relation to the rest of the brain. The evidence is impressive: figure 8.1 shows the relationship between the neocortex ratio and average size of the social group in species belonging to the primate order, including various hominoids, monkeys, and prosimians.

The predominant view seems to be that it was larger group size that stimulated larger brains rather than the other way round, but this strikingly close relationship suggests that our brains are a much more social organ than we usually recognize: they have developed to deal with the demands and problems of social life. This is very much what is implied by the

Figure 8.1: The social brain

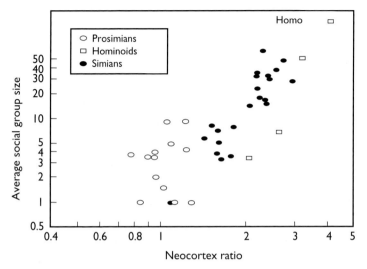

The size of the neocortex in relation to the rest of the brain is related to the average size of the social group among species of primates.

Source: R. Dunbar, "Brains on Two Legs: Group Size and the Evolution of Intelligence," in *The Tree of Origin*, ed. F.B.M. de Waal (Cambridge: Harvard University Press, 2001). Reproduced with permission from Harvard University Press.

analysis presented in this book. We saw in chapter 3 that the main sources of chronic stress in modern societies identified by epidemiological research were three intensely social risk factors: low social status, social affiliations, and early childhood experience. This confirms findings of psychological research, including that from Lassner, Matthews, and Stoney looking at cardiovascular reactivity to social and asocial stressors. They concluded, "[I]t appears that conflicts and tensions with other people are by far the most distressing events in daily life in terms of both initial and enduring effects on emotional well-being" (1994: 69)—more important even than the demands of work, home, and financial difficulties. It also fits with the greater importance of relative incomes and income inequality compared to absolute living standards in modern affluent societies; both suggest that the social meaning of income and expenditure count for more than the goods in themselves.

The fact that our brains have evolved to solve social problems reflects what we have said about the overriding need to negotiate our way successfully through the opportunities for cooperation and potential for conflict with others if we are to gain access to scarce material resources and reproductive opportunities. Without a sovereign power to keep the peace, our ancestors had to develop cooperative strategies if they were to avoid the Hobbesian nightmare of "warre of each against all" (Sahlins 1974). Although the "hostile forces of nature" was Darwin's phrase for the environmental factors threatening survival, it was Richard Alexander who pointed out that the primary hostile force of nature encountered by human beings are other humans. He went on to say that our ability to "traverse this landscape, successfully preventing others from violating . . . [our] interests, depends substantially on . . . [our] reputation and ability to maintain a favourable position in dominance hierarchies" (1987: 274).

The social content of our large human brains is not limited to the affiliative and dominance strategies we have discussed such as snobbishness, social exclusion, and downward discrimination, which we use to maintain status, or to the affiliative strategies and psychology of gift exchange and reciprocity. Also crucial to friendship and mutuality are our powers to empathize and identify with others. In addition to their direct effects, these abilities are also essential to the capacity for imitative learning, which is the foundation of a cultural way of life.

Another major social feature of our evolved psychology is our desire to be valued and needed by others. Sometimes seen almost as a spiritual potential for a sense of self-realization in relation to the needs of others, it helps to secure our position as members of the cooperative group. After all, the best way of making sure you are included in the cooperative group and do not risk being ostracized and preyed upon is to do things that other people find useful and value you for. Interestingly, a recent study of the health benefits of friendship found that the main beneficiaries were the givers rather than the receivers of practical and emotional support (Brown et al. 2003).

There is evidence that we are good at assessing whom we can trust and cooperate with and whom we cannot (Frank 1988). Evolutionary psychologists have shown that we watch out for and want to punish social cheaters and free riders who default on cooperation and threaten cooperative systems (Buss 1999).

Underlying everything, of course, is the capacity to infer people's intentions and state of mind from their behavior, as well as our recognition of our existence in the minds of others. We monitor how others see us, and we know ourselves through their eyes. Through our capacity to experience the powerful motivational forces of pride, shame, and embarrassment, we are pushed around by what we think they think of us. These elements suggest the deep psychology of our social evolution.

A particularly nice contribution to an understanding of

our social evolution came from Robin Dunbar (1996), who suggested that the development of language had less to do with the coordination of practical tasks such as hunting and gathering and more to do with social cohesion and the mediation of social relationships. He argued that the main advantage of speech was that it enabled chatting and gossip, which provide a kind of virtual grooming. As we saw earlier, Alison Jolly described grooming as "the social cement of primates, from lemur to chimpanzee" (1985: 207), or, as Byrne put it, "Grooming denotes what we would normally call friendship. Animals that groom together, look after each other . . . and come to each other's aid when they are in need" (1995: 200). Among humans, not only is physical contact essential to development in infancy and early childhood, but touch is used to convey sympathy and support throughout life. However, grooming runs into trouble as a way of making social bonds if there are larger numbers of animals in a group. Studies of primates have shown that the larger the group, the more time has to be spent in grooming. Eventually the time it takes to maintain alliances and ensure one's place in social networks becomes too great. Dunbar suggests that speech provides a much less time-consuming way of solving the same problem. You can chat with several people at once, explain yourself to them, give them your perspective on events and your version of what happened, recruit them to your point of view, and express sympathy and concern for them and their predicaments.

A number of studies have suggested that our reasoning powers have been honed to deal specifically with social reasoning. For example, it has been shown that people are very much better at solving problems when they are expressed as social rather than abstract problems. When a logical problem was posed abstractly using playing cards, only 10 percent of the population got it right, but when what was logically exactly the same problem was posed as a social problem about whether people might be cheating, 75 percent got it right (Cosmides and Tooby 1992). Such a large difference makes it surprising that we can apply our minds to highly technical, abstract, and nonsocial problems at all.

Nor is the social equipment with which our evolution has endowed us confined to our brains and psychological characteristics. It also shows—literally—in the whites of our eyes. Kobayashi and Kohshima (2001) found that human beings are the only primates (of the ninety-two primate species they examined) to have whites to their eyes. Our white "sclera" contrasts sharply both with the color of the skin that surrounds the eye as well as with the color of the iris and pupil at the center. Most primates have brown sclera and brown skin around their eyes. That our contrasting white sclera was selected during the evolutionary processes must mean that it became an advantage for us if others could follow our gaze and make inferences about where our attention and thoughts were directed. Quite apart from its other social uses, gaze following is thought to be particularly important in establishing joint attention (between parent and child) as a basis for learning in early childhood. Interestingly, chimps occasionally have the same genetic mutation, but among them it has not been selected to become universal. The implication is that among all nonhuman primate species it is better to disguise where your attention is directed. Only among humans is it advantageous to reveal it. Presumably the nature of the social environment among nonhuman primates means that it is not an advantage to be better understood. This reflects a profound difference in our sociality and, above all, in the human potential for cooperation. It suggests that levels of cooperation had reached a point where individuals depended less on subterfuge, guile, and cunning to deal with others, and more on their helpfulness. Others' behavior in response to knowing more of your inner world must, on balance, have been beneficial.

That our eyes have evolved to serve as "windows on our soul," to give away clues to what we are thinking about and where our attention is, is evidence of the long evolutionary roots and depth of human sociality. We actively scrutinize each other's eyes to provide clues to each other's inmost thoughts; we look each other in the eyes particularly to make a personal bond or to help us decide whether or not someone is trustworthy.

The social uses of eye contact and importance of gaze following are matched by the evolution of what are called "mirror" neurons (Wolf et al. 2001; Rizzolatti, Fogassi, and Gallese 2000). These are neurons that fire not only when we do something ourselves, but also when we watch someone else's actions, as if we were making sympathetic imitative movements. As well as these neurons being, once again, important in imitative learning, they are also likely to be part of the basis for empathy and sympathy: perhaps they are involved in making us flinch when we see others hurt, as when watching television or movies. I remember once seeing proud parents watching their sons in a school high-jump competition. As each boy ran up to the jump, a proportion of watchers would involuntarily and unconsciously raise one foot in sympathy at the critical moment when the jumper had to make his leap. Mirror neurons enable a form of identifying with others' actions that simulates being in their bodies and going through their physical movements. This is important in the way we learn by imitation: watching someone else's activity from outside without this sympathetic activation tells us much less than we learn from imaginatively inhabiting his or her movements as if from inside.

Most of this deep sociality is of course completely ignored in public policy—ignored when trying to understand what goes wrong, and ignored in decisions about the economic and social development of our society. Worse than that, when people are treated merely as self-interested consumers, it is more than just ignored. While we conceive of ourselves primarily as self-interested individuals motivated by an asocial acquisitiveness, the danger is that we will so surround ourselves with systems of sticks and carrots, incentives and deterrents, that we will create a misunderstood and unhappy version of the humanity we plan for. We will fail to recognize that what really matters to us, the source of our real satisfaction or dissatisfaction, just like the main sources of our stress and unhappiness, is to be found in the quality of social relations. The acquisitive behavior that drives consumption is actually far from asocial: it is instead a neurotic expression of our desire for approval and respect—our desire to be valued, which has become distorted into ranking behavior by the inequality and status differences that lead to us feeling graded and degraded (Frank 1999).

I have emphasized indicators of the deeply social side of human nature because it is not as well recognized as the self-interested, antisocial side, which dominates our experience of life and the formulation of public policy in modern market societies. Those who argue that economic activity should be about achieving the "real" goal of ever higher standards of consumption, and suggest that inequality may increase efforts to raise living standards but doesn't matter in itself, have failed to understand what is important to us as social beings. Now that the vast majority of the populations of developed countries no longer face hunger or shortages of basic necessities, the modern runaway growth of consumption, which so seriously threatens the environment, reflects how deep our neurotic responses to inequality can go. Too often our social needs appear simply as a mysterious, vague, and irrational part of our makeup, arising either from an emotional and psychological weakness or from a flimsy moralistic ideology.

We should not forget that although dominance behavior is so prominent in modern affluent societies, it does not mean that we must inevitably live in dominance hierarchies. The fact that we struggle for status (or at least to maintain a degree of respectability) when we find ourselves living in a dominance hierarchy does not mean that we must be kept permanently in a dominance hierarchy. That is like saying that because a drowning man struggles to keep his head above water, he needs to be kept in water. Our capacity for more sociable forms of organization is clear not only from an understanding of our social strategies, but also from the record of egalitarianism in our prehistory and from the evidence (in chapters 2 and 4) of how responsive behavior is to small differences in inequality.

We must never lose sight of the fact that we have built-in equipment both for the highly social strategies of interaction usually associated with equality and for the antisocial strategies of dominance behavior. We use both strategies in different areas of our lives—depending on the circumstances. More unequal social environments increase concern for social status and lead to an emphasis on dominance behavior, including more downward discrimination—so contrasting sharply with the more inclusive and affiliative strategies associated with greater equality.

Social Development and Early Experience

As well as the influence of the current social environment, there are of course also individual differences in how affiliative, aggressive, or authoritarian people are. Although there are likely to be genetic contributions to these individual differences, they bring us back to the importance of the programming of stress responses in early childhood that we discussed in chapter 3. We saw that maternal stress in pregnancy and the stressfulness of life in early childhood have life-long effects on levels of stress hormones and so on health. These links are simply the biological side of what developmental psychologists such as John Bowlby have always told us about the lasting psychological effects of early childhood experience. But rather than regarding children who are insecure and have had a difficult early life simply as damaged, it would probably be more accurate to think of a period of particular sensitivity to the nature of social experience as preparing us for the kind of social environment in which we are likely to have to operate as adults.

To fit into any particular society, it is important to have the optimal balance in our social repertoire between affiliative behavioral strategies, on one hand, and the timidity, fear, and aggression appropriate to ranking systems, on the other. But rather than the balance being genetically fixed once and for all, the period of early sensitivity allows the hormonal influences on social behavior to be adjusted in the light of early experience. We need to be biologically prepared for the particular character of social life; as Kemper put it, "It is important that power-status outcomes, emotions, and neurophysiological and autonomic systems are firmly bound together" (1988: 308).

The relationship between early experience and later social behavior has often been seen as a process by which people's relationship to societal authority is modeled on their childhood relationship to parental authority. This comes close to the idea that the function of early sensitivity is to use early social experience as an indicator of the nature of the social relationships we will have to deal with later in life: preparing us to be more or less confident, secure, aggressive, friendly, dependent, independent, trusting, or suspicious. Because societies differ so much, we need a system for adapting and preparing our behavior, emotions, and hormonal responses to local conditions.

In modern societies, where children grow up in a nuclear family environment in which the quality of social relations might be quite different from those in the wider society, the results of early sensitivity can often look counterproductive. Many children are brought up amid great conflict and end up lacking the social skills, such as the ability to trust and cooperate, that are helpful during adult life in modern societies. Others grow up in a very secure and caring emotional atmosphere that leaves them ill-prepared for a world in which personal ambition, competition, wealth, and position count for so much. But in the small groups in which our prehuman and prehistoric human ancestors lived, there was rarely such a sharp distinction between the separate social worlds of the nuclear family and the wider society as there is in modern societies. In the small foraging bands of our prehistory there was less scope for a mismatch between the social environment of childhood and adulthood. Rather than being brought up in separate nuclear families providing self-contained emotional environments distinct from the rest of society, children would have had direct exposure to the kind of community they would have to live in as adults.

Despite sometimes appearing dysfunctional in modern societies, the fact that we have evolved so that early experience has such an important influence on later social behavior is an indication of just how important it is to get one's social strategies right. Given the huge variations in the kind of societies our human and prehuman ancestors have lived in, it is not difficult to see why our behavior might benefit from some early in situ programming or tuning. What is perhaps more surprising is that the effects of early experience are not confined to humans but seem to be broadly similar across a wide range of mammalian species. Even rats that are handled daily between birth and weaning grow up to have lower levels of stress hormones, a pattern that lasts into their old age (Meaney et al. 1988; Vallee et al. 1997; Anisman et al. 1998). Handled rats are better at learning their way through mazes in rat old age. After the discovery of this effect, it was found that early handling is beneficial because when the young rats are returned to their mothers, their mothers lick them more, so it would be more accurate to say that it was an effect of maternal licking rather than of human handling (Liu et al. 1997; Caldjia, Diorioa, and Meaney 2000). The lifelong effect of the quality of mothering is clearly not confined to humans.

Again like humans, in a wide range of mammalian species prenatal maternal stress has long-term effects on offspring very much like the effects of postnatal stress. The sensitive periods start in utero and continue into childhood. Effects of maternal stress in pregnancy have been shown among rodents and various nonhuman primates, as well as among some farm and pet species (Braastad 1998). Several biological pathways linking maternal stress to fetal development have been identified among humans, including a correlation between maternal and fetal cortisol levels (Gitau et al. 1998; Teixeira et al. 1999; Wadhwa et al. 1996). In effect, the tuning of the offspring's stress responses benefits not only from its experience in infancy, but also from its mother's experience during pregnancy. (In addition, insofar as the mother's physiology is affected by the cumulative impact of her lifetime experience, this may also impact the child during pregnancy.)

Although there is some evidence that chimpanzees are capable of different forms of social organization (Power 1991), the young of most mammalian species do not have to be ready to cope with nearly such wide differences in social organization as exist between human societies. Why, then, do they show a similar period of early sensitivity? Part of the answer is that the optimal social and reproductive strategy will vary according to social status. However, it may also be that social organization among many species is much less fixed than we imagine. For instance, as periods of food scarcity come and go, they have effects not only on social organization and dominance behavior but also on reproductive strategies. Food shortages are a common stressor that usually affect both social behavior and reproductive strategies. But exactly what the effects are will vary from species to species. Is it better during periods of hardship to have more young with less investment in each, or to have fewer—or none—until times improve? Is it best to become more aggressive, or to conserve resources and become less so?

Margaret Power (1991) pointed out important differences in the reproductive strategies and extent of dominance behavior among chimpanzees according to whether they were moving through the forest in separate small groups, or whether they had congregated in larger groups around the feeding stations observers had set up make it easier to study their behavior. Robert Sapolsky (1998) reported changes in social behavior among baboons during a period of drought. Often the optimal strategies will vary by social status.

An important indication that the function of our early sensitivity to the social environment is indeed to prepare our responses for the kind of social environment we will have to deal with in adult life comes from the effect of early stress on reproductive strategies. Both early stress and whether fathers are present or absent seem to change reproductive behavior in humans. Teenage pregnancy rates, like violence among young men, are among the clearest statistical indicators of the social damage of inequality and low social status (Pickett and Wilkinson, forthcoming). Within countries they mark out the areas of high relative deprivation, and internationally they mark out the countries with high levels of income inequality. There is evidence that girls who have had a stressful early life are likely to reach sexual maturity at a younger age (Coall and Chisholm 2003; Moffitt et al. 1992). Girls are also likely to become sexually active and become pregnant earlier if they are brought up without a father (Flinn et al. 1996). Perhaps being brought up without a father signals to girls that the social system they are born into is not one in which it is worth waiting for a husband who will share the parental investment in children. Not only do these factors seem likely to contribute to the very strong association between deprivation and teenage pregnancy (as strong as the connection between deprivation and violence among males) but, as Chisholm and colleagues (2001) have suggested, they seem likely to reflect a shift in reproductive strategy. Despite calling it a "strategy," it results of course more from hormonal prompting than from any conscious consideration. If conditions are tough (but not too tough to maintain reproduction), it is better to breed early and often, putting less investment into each child. In contrast, if conditions are easier, it is better to wait until you have a partner, and then make larger investments in fewer children. Essentially it is a matter of adjusting the balance between quantity and quality of offspring to suit the circumstances.

Although we discussed the relationship between violence and inequality in terms of disrespect (chapter 5), the link also reflects the tendency for inequality to increase early stress and its later effects. One effect of early stress is to increase risk-taking among young men. The underlying nature of this connection is suggested by the fact that similar adaptations are also seen among some nonhuman primates. Mehlman and colleagues (1995) concluded their study of macaques by saying that the adolescent males with low serotonin (the hormone associated with social status) "are at risk for exhibiting more violent forms of aggressive behavior and loss of impulse control as evidenced by greater risk-taking during movement through the forest canopy." If low-status males with little or no access to females are to avoid "a one-way road to genetic nothingness" (Pinker 1998: 498), they may have to be aggressive and adopt high-risk strategies. Among humans, it is not only clear that rates of violence are much higher among young men in deprived areas, but accident rates and other forms of behavior that reflect risk-taking also have a particularly pronounced social gradient.

The lasting effects of early stress, often indicated by poor attachment, loss of a parent, and domestic conflict are well-established. More recently a clearer picture has begun to emerge of the hormonal links which parallel the behavioral and psychological ones—how early stress raises cortisol levels and increases behavioral problems (such as hyperactivity), tending to make people more aggressive, less affiliative, and more likely to perceive others as threatening (Raine et al. 1997; Flinn et al. 1996; O'Connor et al. 2002; Suomi 1991; McCord 1984; Gunnar 1998; Visconti et al. 2002; Chen and Matthews 2001).

Though Christopher Lasch (1977) referred to the family as a "haven in a heartless world," its isolation and financial and social insecurity often make it a focus of more, rather than less, stress and interpersonal conflict than the wider world. The growth of inequality that affected so many countries in the last quarter of the twentieth century saw rapid increases in the proportion of children living in relative poverty (Kangas and Palme 1998). Living in relative poverty inevitably increases the stresses and strains of family life. The research suggests that it leads to less "maternal warmth" and more authoritarian and controlling parenting styles (Leventhal and Brooks-Gunn 2000; Earls, McGuire, and Shay 1994; Baumrind 1972). Figures from the Luxembourg Income Study show that the United States and Britain were not only the most unequal of developed countries, but that they also had among the highest rates of relative poverty among children. In both countries a quarter or more of all children lived in households on less than half the national average income (Bradshaw 2000). Some of the grosser effects of increased maternal stress on early life are of course shown by the international analyses of the relationship between income inequality and infant mortality (Hales et al. 1999; Wennemo 1993; Waldmann 1992; Lobmayer and Wilkinson 2000).

The Biology of Stress and Its Impact on Health

The concluding part of this chapter provides a brief outline of the biological effects of stress and explains how it comes to exert such a powerful effect on physiological health. The three intensely social sources of stress discussed in chapter 3 (having a difficult start in life, low social status, and having few friends) point to our central vulnerability to the social world. They reflect our anxieties and insecurities about ourselves in the eyes of others—whether we are interesting, attractive, and capable, or whether people find us boring, stupid, unattractive, gauche, and so on. The question is, how does this get under the skin to affect physical health and longevity?

The central biological mechanisms triggered by stress are those that prepare us for fight or flight. The physiological response to stress involves a diversion of resources and a major shift in physiological priorities. Top priority goes to mobilizing energy for muscular activity. When survival depends on alertness, reaction times, and the ability to run fast, all resources are devoted to that end, and the various biological housekeeping functions—such as tissue maintenance and repair, immunity, growth, digestion, and reproductive processes—are down-regulated.

In our evolutionary past, as in the lives of most animals, emergencies usually lasted for less than an hour, and the diversion of resources from health maintenance processes was too short to matter. A fight, or escaping from one, usually involved only a few minutes of real physical exertion. After the emergency was over, breathing and heart rate, like other physiological processes, would gradually return to normal. The problems arise when we remain under stress, feeling anxious or worried, for weeks or months or years. The shift in priorities as our bodies remain on the alert, in a state of physiological arousal, starts to tell on our health. So broad are the range of possible health consequences that chronic stress can be regarded as acting as a general vulnerability factor, increasing our vulnerability to such a wide range of diseases that its effects have been likened to more rapid aging.

Because so many diseases are more common among the less well-off, Marmot, Shipley, and Rose (1984) suggested that the explanation for health inequalities may involve some factor which lowered resistance and made people less resilient to a wide spectrum of diseases. Chronic stress seems to be such a factor. This is an important point. Instead of thinking of health simply in terms of piecemeal exposure to infectious agents or to any other environmental hazards, we need instead to think more about what affects the body's defenses and weakens its ability to withstand the potentially harmful exposures it encounters.

The broad outlines of the biological response to stress are common to most mammals. The body is prepared to fight or flee by both the nervous system and the endocrine system (which secretes hormones directly into the bloodstream). The autonomic nervous system is, as its name suggests, the branch of the nervous system that controls many of the biological processes that go on automatically, distinct from the branch that enables us consciously to control our muscular activity and movement. Within the autonomic nervous system there are again two main branches: the sympathetic and parasympathetic. The sympathetic nervous system is linked to all the major organs, as well as having a fine network controlling blood vessels, sweat glands, etc. When activated, it causes the release of epinephrine (adrenaline) and norepinephrine (noradrenaline), which contribute to the body's arousal and readiness. Epinephrine is released into the bloodstream by the adrenal glands, and norepinephrine is produced at the sympathetic nerve endings all over the body. The sympathetic nervous system produces the almost instantaneous response that leaves you tingling after a sudden shock such as a near miss when driving.

In contrast, the parasympathetic nervous system is deactivated under stress and activated in periods of relaxation and during sleep. It promotes energy storage, digestion, growth, and other housekeeping or body-maintenance functions. Whereas the sympathetic nervous system increases the heart rate, raises blood pressure, and diverts blood to the muscles, the parasympathetic nervous system slows the heart down, diverts blood away from muscles, and gives priority to other system-maintenance processes. The contrast between the functions of these two branches of the autonomic nervous system is so great that to activate them both together would be like accelerating and braking simultaneously.

The endocrine contribution to arousal also involves the adrenal glands (so called because they sit above each kidney), but it works a little more slowly than the sympathetic nervous system, taking minutes rather than fractions of a second to release stress hormones into the bloodstream. Signals from the hypothalamus (in the brain), relayed by the pituitary (just under brain), cause the adrenal glands to release cortisol into the bloodstream—the so-called hypothalamic-pituitary-adrenal (HPA) axis. Cortisol is the most important endocrine hormone involved in preparing the body for sustained physical activity in meeting a threat. To make energy available, it raises blood sugar levels by counteracting the effects of insulin (which would otherwise make the body store energy), releasing fatty acids from the body's fat deposits into the bloodstream. Cortisol also acts in the brain to increase vigilance, reinforcing the effects of epinephrine. In addition, the pituitary releases a number of other hormones during stress, including prolactin—which serves to inhibit reproductive processes—and some morphinelike painkillers, some of which are also produced by the brain. Much of this makes obvious sense as part of an evolved adaptive strategy that gives priority to dealing with short-term threats and emergencies.

Other physiological responses to stress that contribute to the general shift in biological priorities to meet some threat include the inhibition of growth hormone and of reproductive hormones such as estrogen, progesterone, and testosterone, as well as the inhibition of insulin. Particularly important for its health implications is that sustained stress is also known to disrupt various aspects of the immune system—mainly through the HPA axis but also as a result of the activation of the sympathetic nervous system. In the very short term, immune function is briefly enhanced, but prolonged stress (lasting for more than about an hour) causes it to be down-regulated, making us more vulnerable to infection. One of the effects of chronic stress is the tendency for high levels of cortisol to shrink the thymus gland, halting the production of new lymphocytes, which are crucial to immunity. This effect is so reliable that the size of the thymus gland was used as an indication of long-term exposure to stress before cortisol levels could easily be measured directly.

The increased risks to health, which are incurred when anxiety and physiological arousal are sustained or recur very frequently over weeks, months, or years, are not, however, all due simply to the direct effects of changed physiological priorities. Part of the damage is done by a tendency for the feedback mechanisms—which should return systems to normal values after arousal—to be impaired when they are kept outside normal values for sustained periods. The regulation of cortisol levels is an example. The neurons in the hippocampus that provide the feedback sensors for the regulation of cortisol levels become damaged by frequent high levels of cortisol. Their numbers decline during aging and decline faster as a result of chronic arousal (Sapolsky 1996). This means that the feedback mechanism controlling cortisol levels becomes blunted over the years. Cortisol responses to emergencies are also dulled: instead of reaching a brief peak and then falling rapidly back to normal when the emergency is over, they rise more slowly and take longer to return to what has become a higher normal baseline.

Similar processes are likely to contribute to the up-regulation of a number of other systems involved in physiological arousal, perhaps including the rise in blood pressure and blood-clotting mechanisms with age. If stress, which normally leads just to a transient rise in blood pressure, is frequent and prolonged, it may also alter the regulation mechanisms, and thus contribute to the rise in blood pressure with age.

Interestingly, the tendency for normal blood pressure to rise with age seems to be related to social changes associated with long-term economic development: it is absent in pre-agricultural societies (Waldron et al. 1982) as well as in some modern closed monastic communities (Timio et al. 1988) but becomes increasingly apparent at successive stages of economic development. As well as the rise in basal levels, blood pressure can also show the pattern of blunted responses to short-term stress found for cortisol among the chronically stressed (Kristenson et al. 1998).

The way immunity is affected by chronic stress may, it has been suggested, be part of a related pattern. Because overactivation of the immune system leads to autoimmune diseases, it would be dangerous for the initial heightened immune responses during short-term stress to be maintained. Sapolsky suggests that the dampening secondary effect of cortisol on the immune system may have evolved to ensure that immune responses were soon returned to a normal level of activation. However, when arousal is sustained for long periods, these secondary effects can suppress immune functioning so that it falls substantially below normal levels, thereby increasing the risks of infectious disease.

Another example of chronic stress damaging a regulatory system may be insulin resistance, which leads to diabetes. In the presence of high levels of cortisol, fat cells become less sensitive to the insulin signal to store the energy circulating in the bloodstream.

The accumulated physiological costs of these secondary effects of chronic stress have been called "allostatic load." The term is used to refer to the long-term physiological changes resulting from exposure to chronic arousal. It is marked by higher basal cortisol levels, higher blood pressure, increased insulin resistance, increased tendency for blood clots, abdominal obesity, and suppressed immune function, among other problems. The higher the load, the greater the risks of cardiovascular disease, cancer, and infection, and the faster the decline in mental functioning in old age. (The hippocampus, which is so sensitive to cortisol and harmed by sustained high levels, is central to learning and memory.)

A particularly important pathway to disease involves the more rapid clogging of the arteries, which increases the likelihood of heart attacks. If the energy resources mobilized during physiological arousal—that is, the fatty acids released from fat tissue into the blood—are not used in physical activity, then they are likely to increase cholesterol deposits, which clog the arteries. Hence sustained inactivity and anxiety add to the risks of cardiovascular disease.

The pathological changes caused by chronic stress obviously contribute to disease through numerous pathways, many of which are only beginning to be understood. This is particularly true now that infectious agents are thought to contribute to the initiation or promotion of a number of diseases—such as coronary heart disease and some cancers—that are not normally regarded as infections in themselves. Aging and increased allostatic load obviously have a number of features in common. The effects of chronic stress include what looks like increased wear and tear on some biological systems. Just as aging increases the risk of a wide range of diseases, so too does chronic anxiety. As a general vulnerability factor, it therefore has one of the characteristics needed to explain why such a wide range of diseases are more common among lower socioeconomic groups. However, the existence of a general vulnerability factor does not mean that there are not important contributions from exposure to many specific risk factors as well. Rather, the two are likely to act together, making people more vulnerable to the disease-causing agents to which they are exposed. The results of Cohen's experiment, described in chapter 3, is an example of this. He demonstrated that people with friends in few areas of life were over four times more likely to develop colds when given exactly the same measured exposure to infection (administered as nasal drops containing cold viruses) as people with friends in many areas of their lives (Cohen et al. 1997). Similarly, exam stress has been shown to slow wound healing among students (Marucha, Kiecolt-Glaser, and Favagehi 1998). In addition, several observational studies have also suggested that poorer people are more likely to get lung cancer from smoking any given number of cigarettes than richer people.

The physiology of stress makes good evolutionary sense when the advantages of a more effective response to short-term emergencies outweighed the long-term health costs. But do they always make sense? There is no problem when emergencies are brief and not too frequent, but what about the low-status animals in dominance hierarchies who are often stressed throughout their lives? Even for them, an up-regulation of basal levels of arousal, making them permanently readier to avoid attacks from more dominant animals, would be an advantage despite accumulating health costs. Being more alert to danger and faster to retreat may, perhaps in combination with changes in reproductive strategy, increase reproductive success. The balance of advantage would also be helped by the fact that some of the health effects of chronic stress, such as increased wear and tear, would have their impact mainly in later life, after reproduction.

Although most components of the stress response system seem to be widely shared among mammals, including a period of special sensitivity early in life, the same hormones can produce different effects in different species. So a hormone that seems to increase aggression in one species can sometimes do the opposite in another. In evolutionary terms, hormones, which act as chemical messengers, are difficult to develop because their function depends not only on the development of a gland to produce the hormone, but also on a receptor to receive the chemical message and produce the appropriate response. Once developed, the duo of hormone and receptor tends to survive over long evolutionary time periods, despite huge change elsewhere in the body and in the wider social and material context in which it operates. It is rarely, if ever, an advantage to lose the communication link between hormone and receptor, even though the uses to which it is put may change. Take two examples: first serotonin, which is associated with high social status among many nonhuman primates. Astonishingly, it also affects dominance and submission responses in crayfish (Yeh, Musolf, and Edwards 1997). It seems that its social function has remained broadly similar from the time when crayfish and humans last had a common ancestor, even though dominance behavior in crayfish is a matter of how they make tail flips—quite different from how monkeys show dominance and subordination. A second example is prolactin, which stimulates milk production in mammals, including humans. But the same hormone stimulates pigeons to produce "pigeon milk," which both male and female parents regurgitate from their crops to feed their young. Once again, the function—nurturing young—is the same in both cases, but the physiological processes triggered by prolactin to feed the young have changed beyond all recognition. Apart from their intrinsic interest, the point of mentioning these bizarre examples is that the way the same hormones influence behavior varies very substantially from one species to another. Serotonin may make some animals more aggressive and others less, and although there is widespread evidence among mammals of a sensitive period during early life that tunes later social and sexual behavior, in one species it may make animals more timid, while in another they may become more aggressive—different strategies, but presumably each appropriate to making the best of the social circumstances.

The effects of stress have become particularly visible in the developed world. This is partly because rising living standards mean that the health effects of material privation, poor living standards, and lack of basic necessities are a great deal smaller than they used to be. As a result, the effects of stress are no longer overshadowed by more powerful material influences on health. Second, rather than deaths being common in infancy and fairly frequent at all other ages, the vast majority of us now survive into old age, and when we do die, we die of degenerative diseases closely related to aging processes. This means that, in addition to the short-term effects of stress, the cumulative effects of chronic stress have much more time to make themselves felt. The third reason stress has moved up the health agenda is that, as well as unmasking the influence of psychosocial factors by reducing the impact of material deprivation, economic development has brought other changes to society, particularly the growth of individualism and geographical mobility. As a result, social life has become less supportive and more demanding. It has decreased social support from friends, family, and community and increased our exposure to social status insecurities and other worries about how we are seen.

9

Liberty, Equality, Fraternity
Economic Democracy

Indications of the remarkable power the issues discussed in this book have over us are everywhere. As I write, the current edition of a weekly magazine and the day's newspaper contain the following three stories. First, Pope John Paul beatified Mother Teresa for choosing to be—in his words—"not just the least, but the servant of the least." The view of the poor as "the least" is here almost definitional; there can be no suggestion that he needs to clarify whom he means by "the least." It is not to devalue Mother Teresa's achievements to point out that the beatification also shows that turning one's back on wealth voluntarily and aligning oneself with the poor is sufficiently difficult to be evidence in itself of saintly qualities—presumably because when working with the least, we might be taken for one of them. The second story was about research using an MRI scanner that found that the pain of social exclusion activates exactly the same parts of the brain—the anterior cingulate cortex and right ventral prefrontal cortex—as physical pain does (Eisenberger, Lieberman, and Williams 2003). Remarkably, in this study the pain was not caused by the genuine social exclusion that often goes with lifelong poverty, nor even by the constant experience of being looked down on. Instead, just the hint of an experience of exclusion was experimentally simulated during the course of a computer game. Each study subject was asked to play a computer game of catch with what they thought were two remote—and unseen—contestants using other terminals. The computer was programmed so that after a short time the two other virtual players ceased passing the ball to the experimental subject and passed it between themselves instead. The third item in the press was an article by a well-known journalist writing about his dislike of the "improper" use of English. People's grammar, vocabulary, and pronunciation are often used as an indicator of social position and educational level. As social markers, these are a source of shame and embarrassment—hence the ads for courses to help you improve your English under headings such as "Embarrassed by mistakes in your English?" and the fact that lower-class accents are endlessly parodied by the more advantaged.

Many discussions of equality and inequality suggest we should aim at equality of opportunity rather than equality itself. But even if it were possible to give people an equal opportunity to end up in an inferior position, that would not make it any more tolerable. It is like suggesting that you can reduce the unpleasantness of unemployment while leaving the real rate of unemployment unchanged simply by helping some people to get jobs in place of others. To know that you are fairly allocated to poverty is little comfort and may actually increase the stigma attached to it; it certainly does nothing to reduce the pain of exclusion. The substitution of equality of opportunity for equality of outcome as a political aim reflects a monumental failure even to begin thinking seriously about the causes of our society's problems. Not only does it use an abstract idea of fairness to hide the lack of social analysis, but it ignores the way processes of child rearing, social differentiation, and prejudice reproduce inequality, protecting privilege and passing it from parents to their children.

There can be no doubt of the tendency for social interactions in societies with more income inequality to be more severely infected by considerations of status; by issues of social rank, superiority, and inferiority; and by cults of exclusiveness and celebrity, on one hand, and of social exclusion, prejudice, and downward discrimination, on the other. The increased social tensions are clear enough in the data we have seen showing that greater inequality is associated with a societal deterioration in the quality of social relationships, lower levels of trust, increased violence from those who reject imputations of inferiority, and the effects of increased stress on health. The social pressures worm their way into almost all of us: as greater inequality makes social position more important, worries about one's own rank and performance inevitably increase. Our jobs, status, education, and income come to matter more, and when we doubt ourselves, social contact becomes more of an ordeal, more infused with social evaluation anxieties and fears about how we are seen and how we will measure up.

The analysis outlined in the preceding chapters suggests that the central issue facing modern societies—affecting the health, happiness, and quality of life of all of us—is the quality of social relations. Social relations are built on material foundations. The deep psychology of their structure goes back to the evolutionary importance of how people solve the Hobbesian problem of the potential for conflict over access to scarce resources. The fact that members of the same species have all the same needs means that the potential for competition and conflict within most species is high. How human societies deal with this problem provides the basis of their social structure. The choice lies somewhere between the "might is right" solution at one extreme, where distributional inequalities are a direct reflection of power differentials, and the more cooperative and social solutions at the other, which are associated with something nearer distributional equality. At one end of the spectrum lies the tyranny of dominance hierarchies while at the other are the systems of food sharing and gift exchange of our prehistoric ancestors. All modern societies of course lie at various points between these extremes.

Important in understanding how we relate to these problems is to recognize that we have been living and wrestling with them at least throughout the whole of our mammalian evolution. This has given us a range of very different social strategies and responses that allow us to adapt to the nature of the society we find ourselves in. Where the allocation of scarce resources is determined by dominance, so that the strong and powerful take their fill while the weak wait their turn, then in the same social package will come a range of dominance behaviors—strategies not only for self-advancement (including downward discrimination and prejudice), but also for responding to the invidiousness of being at the bottom. Arising out of that come various male and female sexual strategies reflecting the intersection of considerations of reproductive advantage and of inequality.

Systems of allocation that are not based largely on dominance reflect, to varying extents, attempts to gain the benefits of cooperation and avoid the costs of conflict inherent in dominance and inequality. These bring into play a range of more highly social strategies, including reciprocity, trust, principles of fairness, mutual aid, and an ease of emotional identification with each other. Central is the shift from trying to satisfy our need to be valued through money and status to satisfying it through more directly social sources, which come from knowing that we are valued for the way we relate to people and what we do for them. Cooperative strategies aim to constrain dominance behavior and replace it with more social systems of allocation.

What is obviously true among human beings, as well as among many other primate species, is that both dominance and affiliative social strategies are practiced in varying degrees in all societies. Signs of dominance behavior coexist with cooperative alliances between individuals—usually near equals—bound together by reciprocity. Evolution has equipped most primate species to operate both social strategies in different contexts. In some species cooperative strategies may be confined to close kin, or to alliances and pacts that help with the struggle for status. In others, the balance between social strategies may be struck quite differently, and the whole tenor of social relations is based more on grooming and cooperation than on threat and dominance. But the point is not simply that we, like other primates, are equipped for both strategies. It is instead that where that balance actually falls has varied dramatically from one society to another and from one historical period to the next. In so doing it carries the whole structure of social relations in a society along with it, changing the expression of human nature as it goes. What we are now learning is something of the environmental factors determining where this balance, this expression of our humanity, is struck. By getting the economic foundations right we can, in effect, choose the nature of the social relations which predominate in our society.

The social processes involved reflect a deeply embedded logic or language through which material relations—systems of allocation and exchange—translate into social relations and vice versa. Each form of material relation implies a corresponding form of social relation: the gift implies friendship, market exchange implies the opposition of interests between buyer and seller, and bribes use the psychological power of the gift to produce the obligations of indebtedness. The organization of material life has such powerful social and psychological implications because it keys into primitive mental structures, structures that have been honed to operate the different ways in which we, as human beings, can come together, faced as we are with the huge potential for conflict over scarce resources and the very substantial benefits of cooperation if the necessary social relationships can be established.

Looking at the ground we have covered in the preceding chapters, it is perhaps surprising how much evidence there is of these processes at work in our societies. Take one of the questions used most often (and included in the U.S. government's General Social Survey) to assess levels of trust in a society. People are asked whether they agree or disagree that "most people would try to take advantage of you if they got the chance." We saw that in the countries and U.S. states with more inequality, levels of trust are very much lower (see figures 2.1 and 2.2). Trusting other people means trusting them not to rip you off even if they have the power and opportunity to do so. You can trust only if social relations are based on principles that run counter to and restrain the use of power in the service of self-interest. It is not simply that acquisitiveness, rather than being restrained, is powerfully stimulated by greater inequality and the increased concern for social status; it is also that our understanding of how we are connected to other people changes. In more unequal states, more people at least say that they would do well in a fistfight (figure 7.1).

In many animal dominance hierarchies, the only context in which might is *not* right is in the cooperative alliances that work through reciprocity, mutuality, and fairness. The simplest concept of fairness, and the one that seems to predominate in human prehistory as well as in modern human friendship patterns, is equality. Recent experimental work has shown that even some species of monkey seem to have a strong sense of fairness that, in practice, seems once more to mean equality (Brosnan and Waal 2003). In human prehistory and in modern human friendship patterns, there is ample evidence that friendship and reciprocity are most compatible with equality. It is not simply that human psychology shows patterns reminiscent of some nonhuman primates which may or may not reflect evolutionary origins; it is also that there is a powerful *situational logic* linking social and material relations such that the meanings of one carry over to the other.

At the societal level, no one familiar with the research literature doubts that rates of homicide and violence tend to be higher where inequality is greater. That is perhaps the clearest demonstration that small differences in inequality have social and behavioral effects. There is also substantial evidence from a number of sources (including the work of Robert Putnam) of lower levels of involvement in community life and of trust where there is more inequality. And on the population level, there is now a great deal of evidence that death rates are related to inequality, particularly in infants and adults of working age.

As we have seen, our sensitivity to social hierarchy, to friendship, and to early childhood experience is very widely recognized and has been repeatedly demonstrated. Nevertheless, it is perhaps surprising that these factors are sufficiently important for epidemiological research to have identified them as among the most powerful psychosocial influences on the health of affluent populations. That implies that they are the most powerful sources of chronic stress in modern societies. But why? The answer seems to lie in the fact that the esteem in which we are held in others' eyes matters to us. We want to feel valued and appreciated rather than looked down on and ignored. Social exclusion or imputations of inferiority are painful. The impact of these experiences is neither fleeting nor a sign of undue sensitivity: it is formative.

Liberty, Equality, and Fraternity

Rather than being a new picture, it turns out that these connections are ones that once seemed intuitively obvious. Not only has the social divisiveness of inequality always been recognized, but the dimensions of the social environment toward which social epidemiology is directing our attention are exactly those that have often been the focus of political attention. They were expressed most clearly in the demand for "liberty, equality, and fraternity" raised during the French Revolution and still inscribed on French Euro coins today.

By liberty they did not—despite what life in modern market democracies might seem to suggest—mean freedom of consumer choice. They meant not being subordinate to the arbitrary power of the king, the feudal nobility, and the local landed aristocracy. Overthrowing the holders of arbitrary inherited power was what the revolution was about, and liberty meant not being subject, subservient, or beholden to them. The same concept of liberty was of course fundamental to the American Constitution and to the political writing of Tom Paine, who, like Tocqueville after him, saw American freedom as freedom from domination by landed aristocracy.

The concept of liberty is therefore very closely bound up with the extent of social status differences and the desire to avoid subordination, social inferiority, and dominance. The shame is that what was once the "land of the free" is now more deeply marked by inequality—and the social tensions it brings with it—than any other developed country.

Fraternity directs our attention to the quality of social relations themselves. Using more gender-neutral words, it is easy to see that underlying this demand is the same recognition of the importance of friendship, social networks, and the quality of social relations, which comes up repeatedly in the health literature. They direct our attention to the possibility of social solidarity and more hospitable and supportive social relations which contrast sharply with the dominance relations in more unequal and divided societies.

Equality is, as this book has shown, the precondition for liberty and fraternity. More inequality—of income and social status—creates a bigger problem of relative deprivation and low social status at the bottom. Liberty, in the sense of not feeling looked down on and treated as inferior, is compromised by inequality. And because the dominance relations associated with inequality are inimical to friendship and to involvement in community life, greater equality is also a precondition for good social relations.

This is a neat fit. Epidemiological research on psychosocial risk factors for health is rediscovering what people once recognized as the most important dimensions of the social environment for human well-being and the quality of life. Despite the pleasure of recognizing our discovery as something people once knew, we have to remember that such a rediscovery is only possible because we have become blind to what was once an intuitively obvious truth. We have only to remind ourselves of the passages from Tocqueville—quoted on pages 37–38 above—to see an example of the intuitive grasp of these connections. The French revolutionaries had the same intuitive understanding of it, and so did many of the early socialists, whom Marx called "utopian"—including most of the Christian socialists.

People have recognized the importance of these links almost whenever optimism about the possibilities of change has flourished. This is the direction in which our human social aspirations lean, almost as if there was some primitive memory of an egalitarian prehistory, as if there was a "right way of living" that fits our moral values—a world of fairness and equality, where people have regard for each other rather than seeing others simply as part of the environment to be exploited for their own ends.

From Private Intuition to Public Recognition

Although we have largely lost the intuitive grasp of the social processes it now takes research to rediscover, we are beginning to be able to replace it with something like the first rough scientific outline of the main dynamics of human sociality at the societal level. In effect, the picture that came (or failed to come) simply from our private intuitions is now something spelled out more objectively for all to see in data, facts, figures, and graphs. That paves the way for a conscious recognition of, and public argument about, the outline of our social nature and what kind of society we should try to develop. The research evidence means that the issues can be dealt with more publicly and openly than before. We are no longer dealing simply with a conflict between different people's private intuitions.

The need to understand a wide range of problems facing modern societies in terms of relative income and socioeconomic status is perhaps most simply demonstrated by the fact that although average levels of health, happiness, and well-being in the populations of the developed countries are no longer related to their levels of national income per capita, within each country they are nevertheless all graded by socioeconomic status. Ill health, unhappiness, and low levels of well-being are—like almost every other social problem—more common lower on the status hierarchy, concentrated in the poorest areas.

Figure 9.1 shows the contrast between rises in gross domestic product (GDP) per head in the United States during the period 1950–2002 and the lack of significant improvement in well-being as measured by the Genuine Progress Indicator (GPI). The GPI subtracts from GDP some of the social, environmental, and economic costs our way of life imposes, such as car crashes, pollution, and commuting, and adds in some of the beneficial activities such as parenting and housework which GDP leaves out (Venetoulis et al. 2004).

Much the same picture is provided by other measures of welfare such as the Fordham Institute's Index of Social Health (Miringoff, Miringoff, and Opdycke 1999) or the Index of Sustainable Economic Welfare (Daly and Cobb 1990; Jackson and Marks 1994): they all show little or no improvement despite rapid rises in GDP per head. Even entirely subjective measures, such as happiness, show the same pattern (Frank 1999). Nevertheless, among much poorer countries measures of happiness do rise with economic growth, but they then level off again among rich countries—very much as we saw life expectancy does (see figure 3.1). As Robert Frank says, "Study after careful study shows that, beyond some point, the average happiness within a country is almost completely unaffected by increases in its average income level. . . . [A]verage satisfaction levels register virtually no change even when average incomes grow many-fold" (1999: 111). But within even rich countries there is—as always—a clear social gradient. Again in Frank's words, the "consistent finding" of analyses of "how subjective well-being varies with income *within* a country . . . is that richer people are, on average, more satisfied with their lives than their poorer contemporaries" (112). In short, happiness and measures of well-being in rich countries are more closely related to social status and relative rather than absolute income.

The Social Transformation

During the lives of just a few generations, human societies have been undergoing the greatest transformation our species has ever experienced. I mentioned in the first chapter a photo of my mother as a baby sitting on her grandmother's knee,

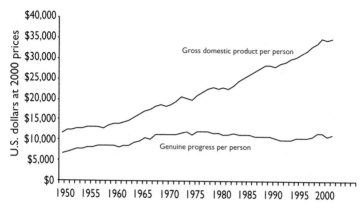

Figure 9.1: Gross domestic product per person compared with the Genuine Progress Indicator per person, United States, 1950–2002

The Genuine Progress Indicator is calculated by subtracting nonbeneficial social, environmental, and economic costs from gross domestic product and adding in benefits, such as parenting and housework, left out of GDP.

Source: J. Venetoulis and C. Cobb, "The Genuine Progress Indicator 1950–2002," available at http://www.redefiningprogress.org/publications/gpi__march2004update.pdf.

and described some of the changes that had taken place during the overlapping lifetimes of these two women, spanning from 1826 to the present. But the pace of change has accelerated: in effect the whole future of humanity is now at stake in our lifetimes.

In the social sphere, rising living standards and economic growth have removed the ever-present threat of scarcity on which the social structures, the dominance patterns and inequalities, of the past were based. As a result, we see all around us the crumbling of the old structures and patterns, but apparently no indication of the character of any postscarcity social system which could give us a sense of the direction in which we are going. However, as we pointed out in the last chapter, we do see what appears to be an almost unstoppable historical trend toward greater social equality, dating back perhaps as far as the beginnings of democracy and the abolition of slavery. Part of the same process is an increasingly humanitarian element in social organization and practice. Despite the appalling and anachronistic counterexamples of our remaining potential for inhumanity that capture the headlines from time to time, a new, more humanitarian ethic shows up in most developed countries in things such as the widespread trend toward the abolition of capital punishment, as well as in the abolition of corporal punishment of children—first in school and increasingly commonly at home. Though racial prejudice is still common, it has lost the intellectual respectability it once had. The same tendencies are also apparent in the development of welfare states, including forms of social security, free medical care, and education.

Although we must recognize our failures and how far we still have to go, it is important to recognize that our emotional ability to identify with each other is broadening, if not deepening. Where once people apparently felt quite unaffected by the suffering of any but their nearest and dearest, it looks as if the boundaries of our moral universe have been expanding: our tendency to identify with each other is slowly spreading from family to class, from class to nation, and now, for some at least, to most of the human race.

Not so many generations ago, torture was not only regarded without a sense of moral repugnance, but also was a normal part of the treatment of wrongdoers. Crowds stood to watch as "witches" were burned alive and criminals beheaded. Now we have laws with huge popular support pro-

tecting even animals from cruelty, and the past looks a bar-
barous place. Although our performance in terms of war and
the prevention of needless poverty-related deaths in the third
world may seem to tell a different story, the trend is for the
armies of many countries to be used increasingly for peace-
keeping and for international agencies to become increasingly effective in monitoring and responding to famine. We
can of course quickly become brutalized, and are still usually
able to burn and butcher people from the air, at a safe distance, but when soldiers are exposed to killing at close quar-
ters, the emotional impact not infrequently causes immediate
vomiting and leaves a legacy of post-traumatic stress disorder.
That there has been a sea change in our sensibilities as well as
in our laws since prisoners were flogged and religious heretics
tortured and burned is undeniable. We appear better able to
identify with each other's pain.

Equally fundamental changes are taking place in other
areas of our lives, including our sexual behavior. Attitudes
have changed toward sex outside marriage, numbers of sexual
partners, same-sex relationships, divorce, sexual expression in
public life, and our willingness to talk about, read, and watch
what would once have been kept private, hidden from the
eyes of others. Insofar as sex was once almost the core of pri-
vacy and private life, this shift in attitudes is part of a growing
erosion of the distinction between public and private spheres.

Despite looking so deep-seated that they might be mistaken for changes in human nature, these alterations in our
emotional makeup are clearly broadly predicated on economic development. That is demonstrated not only by the
historical changes in the developed world, but also by the
broad correlation between levels of economic development

internationally and changing social and emotional behavior. Perhaps social relations, like religious and moral ideas, soften as material life becomes less harsh. Perhaps as our own exposure to pain lessens, we are more affected when we see it in others. Perhaps the extension of our moral universe merely reflects the ever-widening circle of humanity with which we are materially interdependent. Perhaps it is predominantly a reflection of the gentler and supposedly more loving nature of early childhood than was common in recent centuries.

However the links work, the pace and depth of change show how much is at stake in the social development of our species. As humanity becomes knit together in a global interdependence, the basis on which we come together is crucially important. If we are to make good use of the choices before us, it is essential to understand some of the processes that shape our society.

Living with the Market

Partly because of processes such as the trend toward increasing *social* equality, the failure of income inequality to diminish stands out in ever sharper relief. But before moving on to how we might tackle that, there is another obstacle in addition to inequality standing in the path of the development of more sociable societies. It is the unprecedented extent to which our modern material interdependence on each other is organized through the market. We are connected to each other through the self-interested opposition between buyers and sellers. Dependent on our separate incomes, on what is in our bank account or wallet, to maintain respectability and avoid the shame of poverty, we necessarily find other people's needs a threat to our own position and security. Because we feel we need to spend up to the maximum our incomes and credit ratings permit in order to keep up with escalating standards of decency, the cost of helping others financially involves a sacrifice of some of the material security needed to underpin our own social position.

There is of course a sharp contrast between the nature of the practical *material* processes that support our lives and the *financial* accounting and payment systems used to regulate them. In terms of material life, we have become ever more interdependent. Before industrialization, most people were self-sufficient peasants. Each family cultivated its own crops and raised the little livestock it needed for its own consumption. The further back you look in human agricultural history, the smaller the proportion of the things people needed that were bought from others rather than being made domestically. In the course of economic development, this proportion has grown at an accelerating rate: now almost everything we need comes from other people's work, and almost everything we help produce is produced for the use of others. As well as covering a greater part of our lives, this material exchange and interdependence have developed from a local into a global exchange that seems to be turning us into cells in a global superorganism.

The financial rewards and sanctions through which our cooperation is ostensibly motivated seem increasingly at loggerheads with the practical process of our cooperative material interdependence. The danger is that the combination of the market, which emphasizes a very narrow definition of self-interest, and inequality, which harnesses that self-interest to a desire to improve our position in society, tends to make us less social, reducing both our willingness to cooperate and our concern for each other's welfare. Yet wherever the structure of rewards and sanctions appealing to self-interest fails adequately to motivate the detailed cooperative activities of productive life, or gives rise to antisocial behavior, we can only fall back on appeals to the social motivation which the market destroys. The combination of the market and inequality threatens, as we saw in chapter 2, to undermine public-spiritedness and replace it with a tendency to regard other people simply as part of the material environment to be exploited for personal gain. The market produces a less social, sometimes actually antisocial, psychology. The emphasis on a narrow, individualistic self-interest also leads us to try to do no more than fulfill the minimum reward requirements of the market and wage labor, while often leaving us deeply alienated from the real social purposes of work.

We have been able to identify the socially corrosive effects of inequality statistically simply because it turns out that between the opposite extremes of equality and inequality, wider income differences are more damaging than smaller ones. As both Robert Frank (1999) and Juliet Schor (1998) have shown, in the developed world much of the urgency of consumption comes from the concern for social status. Schor has shown that when income differences widened in the United States, savings went down and debt went up, implying that the pressure to consume increased. Indeed, economists have long recognized that how much people save is more closely related to relative than to absolute income. The pressure to consume is also heightened in modern societies because people are geographically very mobile, making us more vulnerable to social judgments that hinge increasingly on external signs and less on more supportive and affiliative modes of interaction. We become easy prey to the invidious social comparisons that advertisers use to make money out of our social insecurities: their success depends precisely on the psychological vulnerability that leads us to seek solace in retail therapy. That we then mistakenly interpret our behavior as evidence of our natural materialistic self-interestedness is a tragedy which shows how deeply caught up in these webs we are.

However, a major role for the market in our lives is still an inescapable necessity. That was the lesson of the failure of the centrally planned economies of the so-called communist or state-capitalist countries of Eastern Europe and the Soviet Union before they embarked on the painful transition to market capitalism after the revolutions of 1989–90. We can of course modify some of the effects of the market by taking whole sectors, such as health care, education, and perhaps public transport, out of it, and we can do a great deal to safeguard people's incomes with minimum wage legislation and good social security systems. We can also limit the extent to which people are exploited for profit, and we can reduce the social damage caused by advertising. But in most areas of life, the modern productive system is far too complicated to arrange for its coordination and integration without buying and selling for profit. Notwithstanding the opposition it creates between buyers and sellers, and the insecurity which comes from our reliance on separate incomes, the price system, which serves to match supply and demand, remains, as economists point out, an important information, coordinating, and signaling system for the allocation of scarce resources of all kinds.

But with smaller income differences and the stronger social

fabric which seems to go with them, the market would become a less exacting force in our lives. The conflicts between the interests of self and society would seem less stark, and God and Mammon less far apart. In a social environment that was less hierarchical, with more genuinely inclusive, egalitarian, and democratic values, we would be less dominated by the market. So although the market will continue to coordinate many areas of life, we can at least partially liberate ourselves from its clutches by reducing the power of inequality that both fuels it and makes it such an irksome taskmaster.

The loss of any belief that there was a viable alternative to the market was a major blow to the political left. Without an alternative to capitalism, it looked to many as if the desire for a more just and sociable society had to be abandoned. But there are, as we shall see, ways in which the social destructiveness and intensity of our experience of domination by market forces can be rolled back.

Reducing Inequality

How can inequality be reduced? The most important issue is political will. As we saw in chapter 6, a 1993 World Bank report describes the growth of equality in eight Southeast Asian economies as having been stimulated by policies designed to deal with crises of legitimacy, often resulting from the presence of communist rivals; governments pursued more egalitarian policies as a way of increasing their public support. We also saw that the British government tried similarly to reduce the social hierarchy during World War II in order to make people feel the burden of war was equally shared in order to gain public cooperation in the war effort. Likewise, in the nineteenth century, Bismarck developed a number of welfare provisions to win public support for his project of unifying the separate German states. From these examples we can see that governments have tended to increase equality not principally when they could afford to but when circumstances provided the political will.

Modern governments are so deeply involved in the economy, often accounting for 30 or 40 percent of economic activity, that they cannot avoid affecting income distribution. During recent decades there have been numerous examples of government policies that have widened income differences and a few that have tended to narrow them. Many different areas of policy can affect income differences, including taxes and social security benefits, education and employment policies, agricultural policies, minimum-wage legislation, the scale of public services, and many more.

Using more progressive taxation to pay for more generous social security benefits may be the most direct way of influencing income distribution; however, such changes are easily undone when another government with a slightly different political complexion comes to power. Although some of the other ways of influencing income distribution may be slightly harder to reverse, they are still highly vulnerable. They also suffer from two other disadvantages: they are imposed from above, and they fail to tackle the root causes of inequality.

Economic Democracy

As well as using the shorter-term strategies, we also need to adopt a longer-term and more fundamental approach to the problem of inequality. We need to make structural changes in modern societies that cannot easily be reversed by successive governments. One way of doing that would be to extend systems of democratic accountability consistent with the market into economic life. So far democracy has penetrated little beyond the election of national and local governments. Most of the institutions in which we work make no pretense to any system of democracy. When we sell our skills and effort on the labor market, we relinquish to employers our control of the uses to which they are put. As a result, economic activity is still controlled by concentrations of economic power that have almost entirely escaped real democratic accountability. People such as Tom Paine, who had such a powerful influence on the American revolution, inveighed against the power of the landed aristocracy and feudal nobility but had no idea that even larger concentrations of undemocratic power could arise through manufacture and trade. At the infancy of capitalism, his failure to foresee the future is easily excused, but our failure to respond to the new accumulations of autocratic power and wealth that now exist all around us is less easily forgiven.

There can be little doubt that we need to push forward the current systems of employee share ownership and find a more democratic and egalitarian way of controlling business. Though most employee share ownership schemes start off simply as systems designed to give employees additional financial incentives and increase their commitment to the company, as soon as employees—or trusts controlled by employees—own over 50 percent of the shares, they are in a position to exercise real control of their company. They can introduce whatever constitution they prefer: they can become a cooperative, they can elect directors, they can have regular democratic policy meetings—whatever they find makes a difference and works.

The relevance of such forms of economic democracy is that they provide mechanisms through which employees can decide on the magnitude of differentials in earnings as well as what happens to profits. And fortunately, such democratic systems are perfectly compatible with the need to maintain a large element of the market in the coordination of economic activity.

Employee stock ownership plans already cover ten million employees in ten thousand firms in the United States with an average employee ownership of 15–20 percent (Gates 1996). Some governments, as in Britain, already provide tax incentives to companies to introduce systems of employee share ownership, and there are a number of tried and tested constitutional systems through which employees can control their workplaces (Oakeshott 2000). In Britain in 1998, share ownership schemes covered 22 percent of all employees and nearly 15 percent of all companies (Conyon and Freeman 2001).

Though a large majority of these systems are intended primarily to provide financial incentives to employees and have very little to do with genuine democracy or egalitarianism, they do take us a step closer to a point where employees exercise effective control. The fact that there are so many firms in the United States in which 15–20 percent of assets are owned by employees makes it a lot easier to achieve (with the help of loans, trusts, etc.) the 51 percent that would give them real control. The fact that such systems were initiated to increase profits should not prevent us from taking advantage of the other objectives they might serve.

Evaluations even of the widespread systems of partial employee share ownership show that the benefits to company performance are sufficiently great to provide a substantial incentive for more companies to go down this road or face being overtaken by competitors. Indeed, there has been a very rapid expansion of such schemes since the late 1980s. Conyon and Freeman (2001) studied the effect on productivity in three hundred British firms not only of employee share ownership, but also of participatory management and profit sharing. They found that each of these components was associated with substantial improvements in productivity. Interestingly, they also found that the results of all three systems together were far better than the separate components on their own.

One of the best-known cooperatives is the Mondragon Corporation in the Basque region of Spain. Over half a century it has developed into a group of over 120 employee-owned cooperatives with 40,000 worker-owners and sales of $4.8 billion U.S. dollars. Mondragon cooperatives are twice as profitable as other Spanish firms and have the highest labor productivity in the country.

Rather than raising questions about whether these institutional structures are compatible with the market, the results of these evaluations suggest the boot is on the other foot: can institutions operating in the market afford not to go down this road? Nor is capital supply a problem: if a cooperative needs more capital than their profits provide, it is free to negotiate loans with banks and others willing to lend at a rate of interest rather than raising money through share flotations.

Companies owned and controlled by employees have transferred control from external share owners, who are likely to have no knowledge or interest in a company other than the profit it makes, to the employees who are the people most intimately involved in it. But would this really make much difference to people's lives, to social relations, and to how hierarchical modern societies are? First, pay differentials would be under democratic control at their source. Where employees elect the chief executive officer, they might still decide to pay that person several times their own wage, but it is unlikely that they would choose to pay twenty or a hundred times their own wage, as happens now, and whatever they did pay would be based on a much more intimate knowledge of the CEO's role and performance. Even when working, as at present, in societies in which huge income differentials are the norm, employees who own and control their workplaces tend to establish much smaller income differentials among themselves. In addition, they presumably regard the income differences for which they have voted as just and fair—not simply in some abstract sense, but in the light of fellow employees' knowledge of what people actually do. And pay differentials brought under direct, local, democratic control could not be reversed by successive governments in the way that changes in taxes and benefits so often are.

If the number of employee-controlled companies increased to become the predominant form of organization, it seems likely that pay differentials would decrease further as societies' values changed. Exceptional contributions of work and commitment from individuals might tend to be rewarded socially (rather than financially) by the appreciation, recognition, and gratitude of other employees. If, at some time in the future, the number of substantial companies that were not owned and controlled by employees dwindled to a small proportion of the total, then the opportunities for the wealthy to command such large unearned incomes would also become fewer. After all, the larger the proportion of a company's shares that are owned by employees, the smaller proportion of the value of employees' work that can be extracted by others as unearned income. And when 1 percent of the population owns 50 percent of the corporate wealth in private hands, employee ownership is also a good way of redistributing wealth.

There are, however, other major benefits of bringing work and economic institutions under forms of democratic accountability. It transforms the status of employees. They cease to be simply the means or tools to fulfill other people's purposes. Instead of selling control of a substantial part of their lives in exchange for pay that reflects power differentials and subordination more than justice, they become people who work cooperatively, as part of a politically equal and democratically controlled community. As such, work has the possibility of becoming an expression of social purpose rather than a demeaning subordination to the will of an unelected and unaccountable employer.

These are changes that represent a very major step toward human emancipation and our failure to make more progress in this direction is scandalous. We know from studies of health in the workplace that people are healthier (with lower death rates) if they have more control over their work (Bosma et al. 1997). Theorell (2004), a pioneer of research in this field, has argued that people reap the full health benefits of having control over their work only if they have a substantial influence over the policy issues that affect their work. (We are now beginning formal evaluations of the health benefits to employees of 100 percent employee buyouts.) More democratic forms of work organization might also be the best response to the substantial body of research showing that health suffers if we feel that the effort we put into work is inadequately rewarded either socially or financially (Kivimäki et al. 2002).

Apart from the productivity benefits, the wider benefits of employment in cooperatives were studied in three Italian towns with different proportions of the labor force working in cooperatives (Erdal 2004). In one of the towns 25 percent of the working population worked in cooperatives, in another 13 percent did, and in the last none did. A general survey of the populations of these towns (varying between forty thousand and eighty thousand inhabitants) found that people thought income differences were very much smaller in the town with more cooperative employment, death rates were lower, social networks were stronger, there was less domestic violence, and the educational performance of schoolchildren was better.

Clearly there are important choices to be made in the way employee buyouts and cooperatives are established and in the ways democratic constitutions work. But there are now many sources of advice, and a wealth of experience, suggesting that the most enduring forms are ones in which each company is owned wholly or substantially collectively, using a trust or cooperative structure (Oakeshott 2000). As well as the support and expertise that ought to be (but usually isn't) forthcoming from the trade unions, governments have an important part to play in assisting this transition, not only by providing tax incentives and capital guarantees, but also by establishing the infrastructure that would ease the problems of industrial restructuring and changes in employment patterns it causes. Providing this support should become one of the hallmarks of all progressive political parties.

A reliance simply on governmental power to redistribute income has often been resented: it too easily appears as the use of autocratic power to take away the pay people regard as legitimately theirs. However, by dealing with these problems democratically at source, we no longer need to look to governments as the primary means of increasing equality. It then becomes harder to paint the development of greater equality as conflicting with freedom. The failure of the centrally planned economies of Central and Eastern Europe and the Soviet Union was a failure of state-owned and -controlled industry. Replacing the market and private ownership of the productive system with state control involved a massive increase in governmental power, far beyond that of governments in Western countries. In contrast, rather than centralizing power, an increase in the number of democratic, employee-run companies represents a move in exactly the opposite direction: a devolution of power and expansion of democracy.

One of the effects of the communist countries' use of state ownership and control of the economy was that the United States lost its liking for equality: people came to assume equality involved a sacrifice of freedom. The equality for which America once liked to think it stood became an alien concept associated with overbearing state power and a loss of freedom. However, if greater equality resulted instead from people gaining greater democratic control of the institutions in which they work, it would be seen as growing hand in hand with freedom.

The Environment and Third World Poverty

It may seem surprising that a book concerned with inequality *within* countries should scarcely mention the inequalities *between* countries. There are, however, good reasons for thinking that reducing the inequalities within rich countries may be one of the best ways of gaining stronger public support for more generous trade and aid policies toward the third world.

As well as the popularity of the disingenuous cliché that charity begins at home, it is often suggested that governments in the rich developed countries have to choose between spending taxpayers' money either on more aid to poorer countries, or on more generous domestic social security and welfare systems. But this is not how things work in practice. Societies that do better in relation to domestic poverty also do better on aid to the third world. It is not by chance that countries such as the United States, with the widest income differences in the developed world, have the most inadequate public services, as well as giving a smaller proportion of their GNP in aid to the third world while, in contrast, much more egalitarian countries such as Sweden have among the best welfare services and give a much larger proportion of their GNP in aid. Once again, it is not about what countries can afford to do, but about their priorities and political will. It is also clear, despite exceptions, that the political parties and kinds of people who most strongly support measures to alleviate domestic poverty are also among those most likely to support more generous policies toward the third world. Why is this?

The differences in attitudes and values related to these issues are partly an expression of the balance between our tendencies to use affiliative and dominance strategies. Whether people's values and outlook are more egalitarian or more in thrall to authority and hierarchy is part of the fundamental psychological and political divide which the Social Dominance Orientation Scale (Sidanius and Pratto 1999) was designed to measure. We have seen, particularly in the last two chapters, how social distances, measured by the amount of inequality, affect these attitudes: larger income differences shift the balance toward attitudes associated with dominance strategies, increasing all forms of downward prejudice, including classism and racism. This mind-set, generated in the context of the inequalities and divisions within a society, is reflected simultaneously in attitudes both to domestic welfare programs and to overseas aid.

But the experience of hierarchy and social distance is not the only way in which domestic inequality affects support for more generous domestic welfare programs and overseas aid. Because greater inequality increases the social pressures to maximize one's own expenditure, it reduces support for taxation. As we mentioned earlier, Juliet Schor (1998) showed that in a period when income differences widened particularly dramatically in the United States, "aspirational" incomes increased rapidly while savings decreased and debt rose—as if people were experiencing a greater pressure to consume. In her words, "The story of the eighties and nineties is that millions of Americans ended the period having more, but feeling poorer." She said that where people once aspired to lifestyles pegged to about 20 percent above their prevailing standard of living, from around 1980 (when income differences started to widen more rapidly), "[a] shift took place in that comparative process—everyone, especially the entire middle class—began to compare themselves with the top 20 percent of the income distribution." Schor describes how when people were asked in 1986, "How much money would you need to make all your dreams come true?" the average reply was around $50,000. However, by 1994, that "dream-fulfilling" level had doubled, to $102,000, and those earning $50,000 or more felt they would need $200,000. As a result, "[p]eople have to spend higher fractions of their income—or above their income—to reach their aspirational targets," and, inevitably, not only did Americans take on record levels of debt, but the proportion of income saved halved between the early 1980s and the 1990s as spending pressures were cranked up.

There is similar evidence of the futility of the continuing rise in levels of consumption in Britain. Despite incomes three times as high as they were in the 1950s, 57 percent of the population believe that they cannot afford all they need, and 28 percent of people even in the upper income brackets think they spend all their money on goods which they have come to regard as "necessities" (Hamilton 2003).

The effects of status competition on consumption (Frank 1999) make it easy to understand how wider income differences lead to what appears to be a more selfish and consumerist society with less to spare for social security or international aid. It may be that one of the best ways of providing the foundations in the rich countries for more generous aid and trade policies to the third world in the future might be narrowing domestic income differences.

The evidence that the pressure to consume comes substantially from our need to keep up with others fits with the evidence that measures of welfare and of happiness have ceased to rise with continued economic growth in the rich countries. Once rising living standards have liberated us from absolute want, they have comparatively little further to contribute to the real subjective quality of human life. Although people continue to want higher incomes, it is no longer legitimate to treat these individual desires for more money as if they add up to a societal demand for further economic growth. If the desire to be richer is a desire to improve one's standing in relation to others, then there is no net gain to be made from uniform increases in consumption.

Nor of course do uniform rises in consumption reduce the problems associated with relative deprivation. Problems of poor educational performance, health inequalities, drug abuse, and violence cannot be reduced while processes defining substantial proportions of the population as socioeconomically inferior remain untouched. Not only is the pursuit of economic growth the pursuit of an illusory source of happiness, but it incurs very substantial environmental costs. Problems of disposing of waste, increasing levels of pollution, global warming, desertification, and depleted reserves of mineral and other natural resources all look increasingly threatening.

. . . and Finally

What matters in the developed world today is the social environment: it is only by improving the quality of social relations that we can make further improvements in the real quality of our lives. Fortunately, the quality of the social environment is not simply a matter for individual wishful thinking or individual commitment to higher moral standards: it is instead built on material foundations. Practical policies affecting how we run the economy and how the organizations we work in function provide powerful policy handles with which to influence the nature of social life.

The alternative to the destructive pursuit of higher levels of consumption is not stagnation—it is a process of social and technical innovation to serve social and environmental purposes. Not only do we need to heal our societies by reducing the sources of social division that give rise to stigma, violence, stress, and intolerance, but if we are to develop a sustainable level of economic activity, we must prevent status competition from fueling the pressure to consume.

The necessary political action will be forthcoming only as the public understanding of these issues increases. Even if a government was persuaded to pursue radical policies in the face of public opinion, it would not be long before it was out of office and its policies reversed by its successor. In addition, the processes of social and economic change are not primarily controlled by governments: most are the unintended consequences of the actions of vast numbers of people and institutional systems throughout society.

This makes it all the more important to change the wider climate of opinion. That means writing, teaching, talking, campaigning, and persuading. It means recognizing that the transformation in living standards brought about by long-term economic growth has changed everything. The scale of relativities, social comparisons, and the need for status and respect that add to our individual desires for more income cannot be satisfied by a societal pursuit of economic growth. As well as the need to reduce inequality, we need to recognize that increased status for some may belittle others; that the increased wealth of the few is the relative impoverishment of the many. We need to create a public awareness of the fact that improvements in the quality of life now depend primarily on the nature of the social environment, which is best served by tackling the material foundations of social divisions, prejudice, and exclusion. We need also to remember that what makes us sensitive to the environment are the basic social anxieties and worries about how we are seen. Hence, we need not only to tackle national issues of inequality, pay differentials, and "fat cat" salaries, but also to think about the nature of personal interactions and what makes people feel valued and appreciated, rather than put down and ignored. It means addressing the way people are treated in the institutions in which we are involved—in families, schools, and workplaces. It concerns not only issues of social status and inequality, but also the quality of early childhood experience, friendship, and inclusion.

But there is much that governments can do without running foul of the electorate. Particularly in the light of the productivity advantages (Conyon and Freeman 2001) and the importance to health of a sense of control at work (Bosma et al. 1997; Theorell 2004), governments could increase the tax incentives to employee ownership schemes and act as guarantors for loans to support employee buyouts (Oakeshott 2000). They could also encourage new companies to set up as democratically run cooperatives. Given the powerful effects of income differentials on levels of violence and on levels of social capital, they could pursue a wide range of policies designed not only to redistribute income, but also to discourage very wide differentials in market income before redistribution. Publicizing the advantages of these policies would do much to gain popular support and would contribute substantially to the necessary increase in public understanding of these issues.

A contribution to greater equality can also be made by reducing the effect of income differentials on access to essential services such as education, health, and public transport. Access to a range of basic services as a right is likely to increase the sense of inclusion and citizenship. But only as income differences get smaller will the majority of people feel that these services are theirs and worth paying taxes for, rather than feeling they are provided for the poor at other people's expense.

We might also hope that advertising codes of practice could be changed so that ads would not continually emphasize the social meanings of inequality by encouraging individuous social comparisons, appealing to "exclusivity," suggesting that without whatever it is, we are second-rate people, and trying endlessly to create dissatisfaction with what we have and what we are. The fact that many countries were able to exercise similar controls over the nature of cigarette advertising suggest that this would be possible.

In summary, while we must accept the operation of market mechanisms—of buying and selling, rationing by price, resource allocation, and the cash nexus—in many areas of our lives, there are a number of ways in which we can dramatically modify their social effects. The fact that modern societies can no longer live without a substantial role for the market does not mean that we have to put up with most of the social damage it causes. We can dramatically reduce income differentials not only by conventional policies, but also by extending democracy into economic institutions and workplaces; this is an important step in human emancipation. Not only does it give people direct control of the pay differentials within their organizations, but it increases their control over their work and puts them on an equal footing with others. By increasing equality it also helps the development of a proper community life.

Finally, none of this depends on reaching some unrealistic, perfect equality. All the data we have looked at come from existing differences in inequality between developed market democracies or between different American states, and what they tell us, above all, is that even small differences in the amount of inequality matter. But rather than appearing to pursue greater equity because of some abstract commitment to a principle to be imposed on the population, we must make sure it is widely understood that the evidence shows that this is the road to a healthier, less stressful society, with higher levels of involvement in community life, increased social capital, and lower levels of violence. These links are far from mysterious; they are merely a restatement of what people recognized long ago, namely, that the important dimensions of the social environment for human well-being are liberty, equality, and fraternity.

References

Adorno, T.W., E. Frenkel-Brunswik, D.J. Levinson, and R.N. Sanford. 1950. *The authoritarian personality.* New York: Harper.

Albanese, A., H. Hamill, J. Jones, D. Skuse, D.R. Matthews, and R. Stanhope. 1994. Reversibility of physiological growth-hormone secretion in children with psychosocial dwarfism. *Clinical Endocrinology* 40(5):687–92.

Alexander, R.D. 1987. *The biology of moral systems.* New York: Aldine de Gruyter.

Altemeyer, B. 1997. *The authoritarian spectre.* Cambridge, MA: Harvard University Press.

———. 1998. The other "authoritarian personality." *Advances in Experimental Social Psychology* 30:47–92.

Anisman, H., M.D. Zaharia, M.J. Meaney, and Z. Merali. 1998. Do early-life events permanently alter behavioral and hormonal responses to stressors? *International Journal of Developmental Neuroscience* 16(3–4):149–64.

Anzaldua, G. 1987. *Borderlands.* San Francisco: Aunt Lute Books.

Asch, S.E. 1952. *Social psychology.* Prentice-Hall.

Atkinson, A.B., and J. Micklewright. 1992. *Economic transformation in Eastern Europe and the distribution of income.* Cambridge: Cambridge University Press.

Banfield, E.C. 1958. *The moral basis of a backward society.* Glencoe, IL: Free Press.

Barker, D.J.P. 1998. *Mothers, babies and health in later life.* 2nd ed. Edinburgh: Churchill Livingstone.

———. 1999. Fetal origins of cardiovascular disease. *Annals of Medicine* 31(S1):3–6.

Bartley, M., C. Power, D. Blane, G. Davey Smith, and M. Shipley. 1994. Birth weight and later socioeconomic disadvantage: Evidence from the 1958 British cohort study. *British Medical Journal* 309:1,475–79.

Baumrind, D. 1972. An exploratory study of socialization effects on black children. *Child Development* 72:261–67.

Ben-Shlomo, Y., I.R. White, and M. Marmot. 1996. Does the variation in the socioeconomic characteristics of an area affect mortality? *British Medical Journal* 312:1,013–14.

Berkman, L.F. 1995. The role of social relations in health promotion. *Psychosomatic Research* 57:245–54.

Berkman, L.F., and I. Kawachi. 2000. *Social Epidemiology.* New York: Oxford University Press.

Berkman, L.F., and S.L. Syme. 1979. Social networks, host resistance and mortality: A nine year follow up study of Alameda County residents. *American Journal of Epidemiology* 109:186.

Betzig, L.L. 1986. *Despotism and differential reproduction: A Darwinian view of history.* New York: Aldine de Gruyter.

Blakely, T.A., B.P. Kennedy, and I. Kawachi. 2001. Socioeconomic inequality in voting participation and self-rated health. *American Journal of Public Health* 91(1):99–104.

Blakely, T.A., B.P. Kennedy, I. Kawachi, and R. Glass. 2000. What is the lag time between income inequality and health status? *Journal of Epidemiology & Community Health* 54(4):318–19.

Blanchflower, D.G., and A.J. Oswald. 2000. Well-being over time in Britain and the USA. National Bureau of Economic Research Working Paper W7487.

———. 2003. Does inequality reduce happiness? Evidence from the states of the USA from the 1970s to the 1990s. Paper presented in Milan, March.

Blane, D., C.L. Hart, G. Davey Smith, C.R. Gillis, D.J. Hole, and V.M. Hawthorne. 1996. Association of cardiovascular disease risk factors with socioeconomic position during childhood and during adulthood. *British Medical Journal* 313:1,434–38.

Blau, F.D., and L.M. Kahn. 1992. The gender earnings gap—learning from international comparisons. *American Economic Review* 82:533–38.

Bobak, M., C. Hertzman, Z. Skodova, and M. Marmot. 1998. Association between psychosocial factors at work and nonfatal myocardial infarction in a population-based case-control study in Czech men. *Epidemiology* 9(1):43–47.

Bobak, M., and M. Marmot. 1996. East-West health divide and potential explanations. In *East-West life expectancy gap in Europe: Environmental and nonenvironmental determinants.* Edited by C. Hertzman, S. Kelly, and M. Bobak. Dordrecht: Kluwer Academic Publishers.

Boehm, C. 1993. Egalitarian behavior and reverse dominance hierarchy. *Current Anthropology* 34(3):227–54.

———. 1999. *Hierarchy in the forest: The evolution of egalitarian behavior.* Cambridge, MA: Harvard University Press.

Boserup, E. 1965. *The conditions of agricultural growth: The economics of agrarian change under population pressure.* Chicago: Aldine.

Bosma, H., M.G. Marmot, H. Hemingway, A.C. Nicholson, E. Brunner, and S.A. Stansfeld. 1997. Low job control and risk of coronary heart disease in Whitehall II (prospective cohort) study. *British Medical Journal* 314:558–65.

Bosma, H., H.D. van de Mheen, and J.P. Mackenbach. 1999. Social class in childhood and general health in adulthood: Questionnaire study of the contribution of psychological attributes. *British Medical Journal* 318: 18–22.

Bosma, H., R. Peter, J. Siegrist, and M. Marmot. 1998. Two alternative job stress models and risk of coronary heart disease. *American Journal of Public Health* 88:68–74.

Bourdieu, P. 1984. *Distinction: A social critique of the judgement of taste.* Translated by Richard Nice. Cambridge, MA: Harvard University Press.

Bowlby, J. 1947. The therapeutic approach in sociology. *Sociological Review* 39:39–49.

Boydell, J., J. van Os, K. McKenzie, J. Allardyce, R. Goel, R.G. McCreadie, and R.M. Murray. 2001. Incidence of schizophrenia in ethnic minorities in London: Ecological study into interactions with environment. *British Medical Journal* 323:1,336.

Boyle, J. 1977. *A sense of freedom.* London: Pan Books.

Braastad, B.O. 1998. Effects of prenatal stress on behaviour of offspring of laboratory and farmed mammals. *Applied Animal Behaviour Science* 61:159–80.

Bradshaw, J. 2000. Child poverty in comparative perspective. In *Breadline Europe: The measurement of poverty.* Edited by D. Gordon and P. Townsend. Bristol: Policy Press.

Brannen, S.J., R.D. Bradshaw, E.R. Hamlin, J.P. Fogarty, T.W. Colligan. 1999. Spouse abuse: Physician guidelines to identification, diagnosis, and management in the uniformed services. *Military Medicine* 164(1):30–36.

Brodish, P.H., M. Massing, and H.A. Tyroler. 2000. Income inequality and all-cause mortality in the 100 counties of North Carolina. *Southern Medical Journal* 93(4):386–91.

Brosnan, S.F., and F.B.M. de Waal. 2003. Monkeys reject unequal pay. *Nature* 425:297–99.

Brown, S., R.M. Nesse, A.D. Vinokur, and D.M. Smith. 2003. Providing social support may be more beneficial than receiving it: Results from a prospective study of mortality. *Psychological Science* 14(4):320–27.

Bruhn, J.G., and S. Wolf. 1979. *The Roseto story.* Norman: University of Oklahoma Press.

Brunner, E., G.D. Smith, M. Marmot, R. Canner, M. Beksinska, and J. O'Brien. 1996. Childhood social circumstances and psychosocial and behavioral factors as determinants of plasma-fibrinogen. *Lancet* 347:1,008–13.

Buss, D. 1999. *Evolutionary psychology: The new science of the mind.* Boston: Allyn and Bacon.

Byrne, R. 1995. *The thinking ape: Evolutionary origins of intelligence.* Oxford: Oxford University Press.

Caldjia, C., J. Diorioa, and M.J. Meaney. 2000. Variations in maternal care in infancy regulate the development of stress reactivity. *Biological Psychiatry* 48(12):1,164–74.

Caldwell, J.C. 1986. Routes to low mortality in poor countries. *Population and Development Review* 12:171–20.

Caldwell, J.C., and P. Caldwell. 1993. Women's position and child morbidity and mortality in LDCs. In *Women's position and demographic change.* Edited by N. Federici, K. Oppenheim Mason, and S. Sogner. Oxford: Clarendon Press.

Casas, J.A., and J.N. Dachs. 1998. Infant mortality and socioeconomic inequalities in the Americas. Paper prepared for the Pan American Health Organization.

Cassel, J. 1976. The contribution of social environment to host resistance. *American Journal of Epidemiology* 104:107–23.

Centers for Disease Control. 2002. *National Vital Statistics Report* 50(15). Atlanta: CDC.

Chance, M. 1998. Toward the derivation of a scientific basis for ethics. *Evolution and Cognition* 4:2–10.

Chance, M.R.A., ed. 1988. *Social fabrics of the mind.* Hillsdale, NJ: Lawrence Erlbaum.

Chance, M.R.A., and C. Jolly. 1970. *Social groups of monkeys, apes and men.* London: Cape and Dutton.

Chang, C.J., J. Fang, and P.S. Arno. 1999. Infant mortality and income inequality in New York City. Paper presented to the Taipei International Conference on Health Economics, March 25–27.

Channel 4. 1996. *The Great Leveller,* television documentary in the Equinox series. Broadcast September 15, 1996.

Charlesworth, S.J. 2000. *The Phenomenology of Workingclass Experience.* Cambridge: Cambridge University Press.

Charlesworth, S.J., P. Gilfillan, and R.G. Wilkinson. 2004. Living Inferiority. *British Medical Bulletin* 69:49–60.

Chen, E., and K.A. Matthews. 2001. Cognitive appraisal biases: An approach to understanding the relation between socioeconomic status and cardiovascular reactivity in children. *Annals of Behavioral Medicine* 23(2):101–11.

Chiang, T.-L. 1999. Economic transition and changing relation between income inequality and mortality in Taiwan: Regression analysis. *British Medical Journal* 319:1,162–65.

Chisholm, J.S., and V.K. Burbank. 2001. Evolution and inequality. *International Journal of Epidemiology* 30:206–11.

Clark, A.E., and A.J. Oswald. 1996. Satisfaction and comparison income. *Journal of Public Economics* 61(3):359–81.

Coall, D.A., and J.S. Chisholm. 2003. Evolutionary perspectives on pregnancy: Maternal age at menarche and infant birth weight. *Social Science & Medicine* 57(10):1,771–81.

Cohen, M.N. 1977. *The food crisis in prehistory: Overpopulation and the origins of agriculture.* New Haven: Yale University Press.

Cohen, S., W.J. Doyle, and D.P. Skoner. 1999. Psychological stress, cytokine production, and severity of upper respiratory illness. *Psychosomatic Medicine* 61:175–80.

Cohen, S., W.J. Doyle, D.P. Skoner, B.S. Rabin, and J.M. Gwaltney. 1997. Social ties and susceptibility to the common cold. *Journal of the American Medical Association* 277:1,940–44.

Conyon, M.J., and R.B. Freeman. 2001. Shared modes of compensation and firm performance: UK evidence. National Bureau of Economic Research Working Paper W8448. See also M.J. Conyon and R.B. Freeman. 2001. Firm benefits from share-owning workers. *Financial Times,* Mastering People Management series.

Cosmides, L.L., and J. Tooby. 1992. Cognitive adaptations for social exchange. In *The adapted mind: Evolutionary psychology and the generation of culture.* Edited by J.H. Barkow, L. Cosmides, and J. Tooby. New York: Oxford University Press.

Daly, H.E., J.B. Cobb. 1990. *For the common good: Redirecting the economy toward community, the environment and a sustainable future.* London: The Merlin Press.

Daly, M., and M. Wilson. 1988. *Homicide.* New York: Aldine de Gruyter.

Daly, M., M. Wilson, and S. Vasdev. 2001. Income inequality and homicide rates in Canada and the United States. *Canadian Journal of Criminology* 43: 219–36.

Danforth, M.E. 1999. Nutrition and politics in prehistory. *Annual Review of Anthropology* 28:1–25.

Darwin, C. 1872. *The expression of emotion in men and animals.* London: John Murray.

Davey Smith, G., and M. Egger. 1996. Commentary: Understanding it all— health, meta-theories, and mortality trends. *British Medical Journal* 313: 1,584–85.

Davey Smith, G., C. Hart, D. Blane, and D. Hole. 1998. Adverse socioeconomic conditions in childhood and cause specific adult mortality: Prospective observational study. *British Medical Journal* 316:1,631–35.

Davey Smith, G., M.J. Shipley, and G. Rose. 1990. Magnitude and causes of socioeconomic differentials in mortality: Further evidence from the Whitehall Study. *Journal of Epidemiology and Community Health* 44:265–70.

Deaton, A., and D. Lubotsky. 2003. Mortality, inequality and race in American cities and states. *Social Science and Medicine* 56:1,139–53.

Department for Work and Pensions. 2003. *Households below average income 2001/2.* Office for National Statistics, London.

Dobash, R.P., R.E. Dobash, M. Wilson, and M. Daly. 1992. The myth of sexual symmetry in marital violence. *Social Problems* 39(1):71–91.

Donkin, A., P. Goldblatt, and K. Lynch. 2002. Inequalities in life expectancy by social class 1972–1999. *Health Statistics Quarterly* 52:15–19.

Drago, F., F. DiLeo, and L. Giardina. 1999. Prenatal stress induces body weight deficit and behavioural alterations in rats: The effect of diazepam. *European Neuropsychopharmacology* 9(3):239–45.

Dunbar, R.I.M. 1992. Neocortex size as a constraint on group size in primates. *Journal of Human Evolution* 20:469–93.

———. 1996. *Grooming, gossip and the evolution of language.* London: Faber and Faber.

———. 2001. Brains on two legs: Group size and the evolution of intelligence. In *the tree of origin: What primate behavior can tell us about human social evolution.* Edited by Frans B.M. de Waal. Cambridge, MA: Harvard University Press.

Dykman, R.A., P.H. Casey, P.T. Ackerman, and W.B. McPherson. 2001. Behavioral and cognitive status in school-aged children with a history of failure to thrive during early childhood. *Clinical Pediatrics* 40:63–70.

Earls, F., J. McGuire, and S. Shay. 1994. Evaluating a community intervention to reduce the risk of child abuse. *Child Abuse and Neglect* 18:473–85.

Egolf, B., J. Lasker, S. Wolf, and L. Potvin. 1992. The Roseto effect: A 50-year comparison of mortality rates. *American Journal of Public Health* 82:1,089–92.

Eisenberg, J.F. 1981. *The mammalian radiations: An analysis of trends in evolution, adaptation, and behavior.* Chicago: University of Chicago Press.

Eisenberger, N.I., M.D. Lieberman, and K.D. Williams. 2003. Does rejection hurt? An fMRI study of social exclusion. *Science* 302:290.

Elliot, J. 1996. *Blue eyed.* Dir. Bertram Verhaag.

Elmer, N. 2001. *Self-esteem: The costs and causes of low self-worth.* York: Joseph Rowntree Foundation.

Emerson, R.W. 1883. *The conduct of life.* London: Macmillan.

Erdal, D. 1999. The psychology of sharing: an evolutionary approach. Unpublished Ph.D. thesis. University of St. Andrews.

Erdal, D., and A. Whiten. 1996. Egalitarianism and Machiavellian intelligence in human evolution. In *Modelling the early human mind*. Edited by P. Mellars and K. Gibson. Cambridge: McDonald Institute for Archeological Research Monographs.

Fajnzylber, P., D. Lederman, and N. Loayza. 2002. Inequality and violent crime. *Journal of Law and Economics* 45(1):1–40.

Fang, J., C.J. Chang, and P.S. Arno. 1999. Income inequality and infant mortality by zip code in New York City. *American Journal of Epidemiology* 149(11 Suppl.): 204.

Fang, J., S. Madhavan, W. Bosworth, and M.H. Alderman. 1998. Residential segregation and mortality in New York City. *Social Science and Medicine* 47(4):469–76.

Finkler, K. 1997. Gender, domestic violence and sickness in Mexico. *Social Science and Medicine* 45(8):1,147–60.

Fisek, M.H., and R. Ofshe. 1970. The process of status evolution. *Sociometry* 33:327–46.

Flinn, M.V., R.J. Quinlan, M.T. Turner, S.A. Decker, and B.G. England. 1996. Male-female differences in effects of parental absence on glucocorticoid stress response. *Human Nature—An Interdisciplinary Biosocial Perspective* 7(2): 125–62.

Frank, R.H. 1988. *Passions within reason: The strategic role of the emotions.* New York: W.W. Norton.

———. 1999. *Luxury fever: Why money fails to satisfy in an era of success.* New York: Free Press.

Franzini, L., J. Ribble, and W. Spears. 2001. The effects of income inequality and income level on mortality vary by population size in Texas counties. *Journal of Health and Social Behavior* 42:373–87.

Franzini, L., and W. Spears. 2003. Contributions of social conditions to inequalities in years of life lost to heart disease in Texas. *Social Science and Medicine* 57(10):1,847–61.

Fraser, C. 1984. The follow-up study: Psychological aspects. In *Low birth weight:*

A medical, psychological and social study. Edited by R. Illsley and R.G. Mitchell. Chichester: Wiley.

Gardner, P.M. 1991. Foragers' pursuit of individual autonomy. *Current Anthropology* 32(5):543–72.

Gates, G. 1996. Holding your own: The case for employee capitalism. *Demos Quarterly* 8:8–10.

Geronimus, A.T., J. Bound, T.A. Waidmann, C.G. Colen, and D. Steffick. 2001. Inequality in life expectancy, functional status, and active life expectancy across selected black and white populations in the United States. *Demography* 38(2):227–51.

Gilbert, P. 1992. *Depression: The evolution of powerlessness.* Hove: Erlbaum.

———. 1998. What is shame? Some core issues and controversies. In *Shame: interpersonal behavior, psychopathology and culture.* Edited by P. Gilbert and B. Andrews. New York: Oxford University Press.

Gilbert, P., S. Allan, and K. Goss. 1996. Parental representations, shame, interpersonal problems, and vulnerability to psychopathology. *Clinical Psychology and Psychotherapy* 3(1):23–34.

Gilbert, P., and M.T. McGuire. 1998. Shame, status, and social roles: Psychobiology and evolution. In *Shame: Interpersonal behavior, psychopathology, and culture.* Edited by P. Gilbert and B. Andrews. New York: Oxford University Press.

Gilligan, J. 1996. *Violence: Our deadly epidemic and its causes.* New York: G.P. Putnam.

———. 2001. *Preventing violence.* London: Thames and Hudson.

Gitau, R., A. Cameron, N.M. Fisk, and V. Glover. 1998. Fetal exposure to maternal cortisol. *Lancet* 352:707–8.

Gorbachev, M. 1987. "The way ahead . . . more democracy and openness." *The Guardian.* Monday, February 2.

Gorey, K.M. 1994. The association of socioeconomic inequality with cancer incidence: An explanation for racial group cancer incidence. Ph.D. diss., State University of New York at Buffalo.

Grant, L. 2000. Take no prisoners. *The Guardian,* Weekend, May 13.

Gravelle, H. 1998. How much of the relationship between population mortality and inequality is a statistical artefact? *British Medical Journal* 316:382–85.

Gunnar, M.R. 1998. Quality of early care and buffering of neuroendocrine stress reactions: Potential effects on the developing human brain. *Preventive Medicine* 27(2):208–11.

Gunnell, D., E. Whitley, M.N. Upton, A. McConnachie, G. Davey Smith, and G.C.M. Watt. 2003. Associations of height, leg length, and lung function with cardiovascular risk factors in the Midspan Family Study. *Journal of Epidemiology and Community Health* 57:141–46.

Hajdu, P., M. McKee, and F. Bojan. 1995. Changes in premature mortality differentials by marital status in Hungary and England and Wales. *European Journal of Public Health* 5:529–64.

Hales, S., P. Howden-Chapman, C. Salmond, A. Woodward, and J. Mackenbach. 1999. National infant mortality rates in relation to gross national product and distribution of income. *Lancet* 354:2,047.

Halpern, D.S. 1993. Minorities and mental health. *Social Science and Medicine* 36:597–607.

Hamilton, C. 2003. *Overconsumption in Britain: A culture of middle-class complaint?* Discussion Paper no. 57, Australian Institute, Canberra.

Hartmann, P. 1977. A perspective on the study of social attitudes. *European Journal of Social Psychology* 7(1):85–96.

Hemingway, H., H. Kuper, and M.G. Marmot. 2002. Psychosocial factors in the primary and secondary prevention of coronary heart disease. In *Evidence-based cardiology*. Edited by S. Yusef, J.A. Cairns, A.J. Camm, E.L. Fallen, and B.J. Gersh. 2nd ed. London: BMJ Books.

Hertzman, C. 1995. *Environment and health in central and eastern Europe.* Washington, D.C.: World Bank.

Hertzman, C., S. Kelly, and M. Bobak. 1996. *East-West life expectancy gap in Europe: Environmental and non-environmental determinants.* Dortrecht: Kluwer Academic Publishers.

Higley, J.D., S.T. King, M.F. Hasert, M. Champoux, S.J. Suomi, and M. Linnoila. 1996. Stability of interindividual differences in serotonin function and its relationship to severe aggression and competent social behavior in rhesus macaque females. *Neuropsychopharmacology* 14(1):67–76.

Hobbes, T. 1996. *Leviathan.* Edited by Richard Tuck. Cambridge: Cambridge University Press.

House, J.S., K.R. Landis, and D. Umberson. 1988. Social relationships and health. *Science* 241:540–45.

Hsieh, C.C., and M.D. Pugh. 1993. Poverty, income inequality, and violent crime: A meta-analysis of recent aggregate data studies. *Criminal Justice Review* 18:182–202.

Jackson, T., and N. Marks. 1994. *U.K. Index of Sustainable Economic Welfare.* Stockholm Environment Institute in cooperation with New Economic Foundation.

James, O. 1995. *Juvenile violence in a winner-loser culture: Socioeconomic and familial origins of the rise in violence against the person.* London: Free Association Books.

Jefferis, B.J.M.H., C. Power, and C. Hertzman. 2002. Birth weight, childhood socioeconomic environment, and cognitive development in the 1958 British birth cohort study. *British Medical Journal* 325:305.

Jolly, A. 1985. *The evolution of primate behavior.* (2nd ed.) New York: Macmillan.

Jung, C.G. 1917. *Gesammelte werke, vol. 7: Uber die psychologie des unbewussten* (1964).

Kalma, A. 1991. Hierarchisation and dominance assessment at first glance. *European Journal of Social Psychology* 21:165–81.

Kangas, O., and J. Palme. 1998. Does social policy matter? Poverty cycles in OECD countries. Luxembourg Income Study Working Paper 187, September.

Kaplan, G.A., E. Pamuk, J.W. Lynch, R.D. Cohen, and J.L. Balfour. 1996. Inequality in income and mortality in the United States: Analysis of mortality and potential pathways. *British Medical Journal* 312:999–1,003.

Kapur, A. 1998. Poor but prosperous. *Atlantic Monthly* (September): 40–45.

Karasek, R., and T. Theorell. 1990. *Healthy work: Stress, productivity and the reconstruction of working life.* New York: Basic Books.

Karlsen, S., J.Y. Nazroo, and R. Stephenson. 2002. Ethnicity, environment and health: Putting ethnic inequalities in health in their place. *Social Science & Medicine* 55(9):1,647–61.

Kawachi, I., and B.P. Kennedy. 1997. The relationship of income inequality to mortality—does the choice of indicator matter? *Social Science & Medicine* 45:1,121–27.

Kawachi, I., B.P. Kennedy, V. Gupta, and D. Prothrow-Stith. 1999. Women's status and the health of women: A view from the States. *Social Science and Medicine* 48(1):21–32.

Kawachi, I., B.P. Kennedy, K. Lochner, and D. Prothrow-Stith. 1997. Social capital, income inequality and mortality. *American Journal of Public Health* 87:1,491–98.

Kemper, T.D. 1988. The two dimensions of sociality. In *Social fabrics of the mind*. Edited by M.R.A. Chance. Hillsdale, NJ: Lawrence Erlbaum.

Kennedy, B.P., I. Kawachi, and E. Brainerd. 1998. The role of social capital in the Russian mortality crisis. *World Development* 26(11):2,029–204.

Kennedy, B.P., I. Kawachi, R. Glass, and D. Prothrow-Stith. 1998. Income distribution, socioeconomic status, and self-rated health in the U.S.: A multilevel analysis. *British Medical Journal* 317:917–21.

Kennedy, B.P., I. Kawachi, K. Lochner, C.P. Jones, and D. Prothrow-Stith. 1997. (Dis)respect and black mortality. *Ethnicity & Disease* 7:207–14.

Kennedy, B.P., I. Kawachi, and D. Prothrow-Stith. 1996. Income distribution and mortality: Cross sectional ecological study of the Robin Hood index in the United States. *British Medical Journal* 312:1,004–7. See also B.P. Kennedy, I. Kawachi, and D. Prothrow-Stith. 1996. Important correction. *British Medical Journal* 312:1,194.

Kennedy B.P., I. Kawachi, D. Prothrow-Stith, and V. Gupta. 1998. Income inequality, social capital and firearm-related violent crime. *Social Science and Medicine* 47:7–17.

Kiecolt-Glaser, J.K., R. Glaser, J.T. Cacioppo, R.C. MacCallum, M. Snydersmith, C. Kim, and W.B. Malarkey. 1997. Marital conflict in older adults: Endocrinological and immunological correlates. *Psychosomatic Medicine* 59(4):339–49.

Kiecolt-Glaser, J.K., R. Glaser, J.T. Cacioppo, and W.B. Malarkey. 1998. Marital stress: Immunologic, neuroendocrine, and autonomic correlates. *Annals of the New York Academy of Sciences* 840:656–63.

Kivimäki, M., P. Leino-Arjas, R. Luukkonen, H. Riihimäki, J. Vahtera, and

J. Kirjonen. 2002. Work stress and risk of cardiovascular mortality: Prospective cohort study of industrial employees. *British Medical Journal* 325:857.

Kobayashi, H., and S. Kohshima. 2001. Unique morphology of the human eye and its adaptive meaning: Comparative studies on external morphology of the primate eye. *Journal of Human Evolution* 40(5):419–35.

Kramer, P. 1993. *Listening to Prozac.* New York: Penguin Books.

Kristenson, M., K. Orth-Gomer, Z. Kucinskiene, B. Bergdahl, H. Calkauskas, I. Balinkyniene, and A.G. Olsson. 1998. Attenuated cortisol response to a standardised stress test in Lithuanian versus Swedish men: The LiVicordia Study. *International Journal of Behavioural Medicine* 5(1):17–30.

Lantz, P.M., J.S. House, J.M. Lepkowski, D.R. Williams, R.P. Mero, and J.M. Chen. 1998. Socioeconomic factors, health behaviors, and mortality—results from a nationally representative prospective study of US adults. *Journal of the American Medical Association* 279(21):1,703–8.

Larsen, C.P. 1995. Biological changes in human populations with agriculture. *Annual Review of Anthropology* 24:185–213.

Lasch, C. 1997. *Haven in a heartless world: The family besieged.* New York: Basic Books.

Lassner, J.B., K.A. Matthews, and C.M. Stoney. 1994. Are cardiovascular reactors to asocial stress also reactors to social stress? *Journal of Personality and Social Psychology* 66(1):69–77.

Layard, R. 2003. Happiness: Has social science a clue? Lionel Robbins Memorial Lectures, delivered at the London School of Economics, March 3–5.

Le Grand, J. 1987. An international comparison of inequalities in health. Welfare State Programme Discussion Paper 16, London School of Economics.

Leary, M.R., and R.M. Kowlaski. 1995. *Social anxiety.* New York: Guilford Press.

LeClere, F.B., and M.J. Soobader. 2000. The effect of income inequality on the health of selected U.S. demographic groups. *American Journal of Public Health* 90(12):1,892–7.

Lee, M.R., and W.B. Bankston. 1999. Political structure, economic inequality, and homicide: A cross-sectional analysis. *Deviant Behavior: An Interdisciplinary Journal* 19:27–55.

Lee, P.C. 1996. Inferring cognition from social behaviour in nonhumans. In *Modelling the early human mind*. Edited by P. Mellars and K. Gibson. Cambridge: McDonald Institute for Archaeology.

Leon, D., and R.G. Wilkinson. 1998. Inequalities in prognosis: Socioeconomic differences in cancer and heart disease survival. In *Health inequalities in European countries*. Edited by J. Fox. Aldershot: Gower.

Leventhal, T., and J. Brooks-Gunn. 2000. The neighborhoods they live in: The effects of neighborhood residence on child and adolescent outcomes. *Psychological Bulletin* 126(2):309–37.

Levinson, D. 1989. *Family violence in cross-cultural perspective*. Newbury Park, CA: Sage.

Lewis, H.B. 1980. "Narcissistic personality" or "Shame-prone superego mode." *Comparative Psychotherapy* 1:59–80.

Lewis, M., and D. Ramsay. 2002. Cortisol response to embarrassment and shame. *Child Development* 73(4):1,034–45.

Liu, D., J. Diorio, B. Tannenbaum, C. Caldji, D. Francis, A. Freedman, S. Sharma, D. Pearson, P.M. Plotsky, and M.J. Meaney. 1997. Maternal care, hippocampal glucocorticoid receptors, and hypothalamic-pituitary-adrenal responses to stress. *Science* 277:1,659–62.

Lobmayer, P., and R.G. Wilkinson. 2000. Income, inequality and mortality in 14 developed countries. *Sociology of Health and Illness* 22(4):401–14.

———. 2002. Inequality, residential segregation by income, and mortality in U.S. cities. *Journal of Epidemiology and Community Health* 56(3):183–87.

Long, J.M., J.J. Lynch, N.M. Machiran, S.A. Thomas, and K. Malinow. 1982. The effect of status on blood pressure during verbal communication. *Journal of Behavioral Medicine* 5:165–72.

Lundberg, O. 1993. The impact of childhood living conditions on illness and mortality in adulthood. *Social Science and Medicine* 36:1,047–52.

Lynch, J., G. Davey Smith, S. Harper, M. Hillemeier, N. Ross, G.A. Kaplan, and M. Wolfson. 2004. Is income inequality a determinant of population health? Part 1. A systematic review. *Milbank Quarterly* 82(1):5–99.

Lynch, J., G. Davey Smith, M. Hillemeier, M. Shaw, T. Raghunathan, and G. Kaplan. 2001. Income inequality, the psychosocial environment and health. *Lancet* 358(9277):194–200.

Lynch, J., G. Davey Smith, G.A. Kaplan, and J.S. House. 2000. Income inequality and mortality: Importance to health of individual income, psychosocial environment, or material conditions. *British Medical Journal* 320:1,200–3.

Lynch, J., G.A. Kaplan, E.R. Pamuk, R.D. Cohen, K.E. Heck, J.L. Balfour, and I.H. Yen. 1998. Income inequality and mortality in metropolitan areas of the United States. *American Journal of Public Health* 88:1,074–80.

Mahler, V.A. 2002. Exploring the subnational dimension of income inequality: An analysis of the relationship between inequality and electoral turnout in the developed countries. Luxembourg Income Study Working Paper 292, January.

Marmot, M., and M. Bobak. 2000. International comparators and poverty and health in Europe. *British Medical Journal* 321:1,124–28.

Marmot, M.G., H. Bosma, H. Hemingway, E. Brunner, and S. Stansfeld. 1997. Contribution of job control and other risk factors to social variations in coronary heart disease incidence. *Lancet* 350(9073):235–39.

Marmot, M.G., and G. Davey Smith. 1989. Why are the Japanese living longer? *British Medical Journal* 299:1,547–51.

Marmot, M.G., M.J. Shipley, and G. Rose. 1984. Inequalities in death—Specific explanations of a general pattern? *Lancet* (May 5):1,003–6.

Marmot, M., and R.G. Wilkinson. 2001. Psychosocial and material pathways in the relation between income and health: A response to Lynch et al. *British Medical Journal* 322:1,233–36.

Marucha, P.T., J.K. Kiecolt-Glaser, and M. Favagehi. 1998. Mucosal wound healing is impaired by examination stress. *Psychosomatic Medicine* 60(3):362–65.

Marx, K., and F. Engels. 1848. *The manifesto of the Communist Party.*

Mathews, F., P. Yudkin, and A. Neil. 1999. Influence of maternal nutrition on outcome of pregnancy: Prospective cohort study. *British Medical Journal* 319:339–43.

McCall, N. 1994. *Makes me wanna holler: A young black man in America.* New York: Random House.

McCord, C., and H.P. Freeman. 1990. Excess mortality in Harlem. *New England Journal of Medicine* 322:173–77.

McCord, J. 1984. Early stress and future personality. In *Stress and disability in childhood.* Edited by N.R. Butler and B.D. Corner. Bristol: Wright.

McIsaac, S.J., and R.G. Wilkinson. 1997. Income distribution and cause-specific mortality. *European Journal of Public Health* 7:45–53.

Meaney, M.J., D.H. Aitken, C. van Berkel, S. Bhatnagar, and R.M. Sapolsky. 1988. Effect of neonatal handling on age-related impairments associated with the hippocampus. *Science* 239:766–68.

Mehlman, P.T., J.D. Higley, I. Faucher, A.A. Lilly, D.M. Taub, J. Vickers, S.J. Suomi, and M. Linnoila. 1995. Correlation of CSF 5-HIAA concentration with sociality and the timing of emigration in free-ranging primates. *American Journal of Psychiatry* 152(6):907–13.

Mellor, J.M., and J. Milyo. 2002. Income inequality and health status in the United States: Evidence from the current population survey. *Journal of Human Resources* 37(3):510–39.

Messner, S.F., and R. Rosenfeld. 1997. Political restraint of the market and levels of criminal homicide: a cross-national application of institutional-anomie theory. *Social Forces* 75(4):1,393–1,416.

Milgram, S. 1974. *Obedience to authority: An experimental view.* New York: Harper.

Miringoff, M-L., M. Miringoff, and S. Opdycke. 1996. The growing gap between standard economic indicators and the nation's social health. *Challenge* (July-August): 17–22.

Moffitt, T.E., G.L. Brammer, A. Caspi, J.P. Fawcett, M. Raleigh, A. Yuwiler, and P. Silva. 1998. Whole blood serotonin relates to violence in an epidemiological study. *Biological Psychiatry* 43(6):446–57.

Moffitt, T.E., A. Caspi, J. Belski, and P.A. Silva. 1992. Childhood experience and the onset of menarche: A test of a sociobiological model. *Child Development* 63:47–58.

Montgomery, S.M., M.J. Bartley, D.G. Cook, and M.E.J. Wadsworth. 1996. Health and social precursors of unemployment in young men in Great Britain. *Journal of Epidemiology and Community Health* 50(4):415–22.

Montgomery, S.M., M.J. Bartley, and R.G. Wilkinson. 1997. Family conflict and slow growth. *Archives of the Diseases of Childhood* 77:326–30.

Montgomery, S.M., L.R. Berney, and D. Blane. 2000. Prepubertal stature and blood pressure in early old age. *Archives of Diseases of Childhood* 82(5):358–63.

Morgan, D., K.A. Grant, H.D. Gage, R.H. Mach, J.R. Kaplan, O. Prioleau, S.H.

Nader, N. Buchheimer, R.L. Ehrenkaufer, and M.A. Nader. 2002. Social dominance in monkeys: Dopamine D2 receptors and cocaine self-administration. *Nature Neuroscience* 5(2):169–74.

Neapolitan, J.L. 1999. A comparative analysis of nations with low and high levels of violent crime. *Journal of Criminal Justice* 27(3):259–74.

Ng, F., and M.H. Bond. 2002. Economic, social and psychological factors predicting homicide: A cross-national study. Chinese University of Hong Kong.

Oakeshoot, R. 2000. Jobs and fairness: the logic and experience of employee ownership. Norwich: Michael Russell.

O'Connor, T.G., J. Heron, J. Golding, M. Beveridge, and V. Glover. 2002. Maternal antenatal anxiety and children's behavioural/emotional problems at 4 years: Report from the Avon Longitudinal Study of Parents and Children. *British Journal of Psychiatry* 180:502–8.

Office of Health Economics. 1992. *Compendium of health statistics.* London: OHE.

———. 1993. *Briefing: The impact of unemployment on health.* No. 29, July. London: OHE.

Paine, T. *The rights of man.*

Pattussi, M.P., W. Marcenes, R. Croucher, and A. Sheiham. 2001. Social deprivation, income inequality, social cohesion and dental caries in Brazilian school children. *Social Science and Medicine* 53(7):915–25.

Phillips, D.I.W., and D.J.P. Barker. 1997. Association between low birth weight and high resting pulse in adult life: Is the sympathetic nervous system involved in programming the insulin resistance syndrome? *Diabetic Medicine* 14:673–77.

Phillips, D.I.W., B.R. Walker, R.M. Reynolds, D.E.H. Flanagan, P.J. Wood, C. Osmond, D.J.P. Barker, and C.B. Whorwood. 2000. Low birth weight predicts elevated plasma cortisol concentrations in adults from 3 populations. *Hypertension* 35(6):1,301–6.

Pickett, K.E., J. Collins, C. Masie, and R.G. Wilkinson. 2005. The effects of racial density and income incongruity on pregnancy outcomes. *Social Science and Medicine* (in press).

Pickett, K.E., S. Kelly, E. Brunner, R. Leach, and R.G. Wilkinson. 2005 (forthcoming). Wider income gaps, wider waistbands? An ecological study of obesity and income inequality.

Pickett, K.E., and R.G. Wilkinson. 2005 (forthcoming). Teenage births, violence and income inequality.

Pigou, A.C. 1932. *Economics of welfare.* London: MacMillan.

Pinker, S. 1997. *How the mind works.* New York: W.W. Norton.

Plato. 1970. *The Laws.* Translated by T.J. Saunders. Harmondsworth: Penguin.

Power, M. 1991. *The egalitarians, human and chimpanzee: An anthropological view of social organization.* Cambridge: Cambridge University Press.

Prandy, K. 1990. The revised Cambridge scale of occupations. *Sociology* 24(4):629–55.

Pruessner, J.C., D.H. Hellhammer, and C. Kirschbaum. 1999. Low self-esteem, induced failure and the adrenocortical stress response. *Personality and Individual Differences* 27(3):477–89.

Pusey, A., J. Williams, and J. Goodall. 1997. The influence of dominance rank on the reproductive success of female chimpanzees. *Science* 277:828–31.

Putnam, R.D. 2000. *Bowling Alone: The collapse and Revival of American Community.* New York: Simon & Schuster.

Putnam, R.D., R. Leonardi, and R.Y. Nanetti. 1993. *Making democracy work: Civic traditions in modern Italy.* Princeton: Princeton University Press.

Raine, A., P.A. Brennan, D.P. Farrington, and S.A. Mednick, eds. 1997. *Biosocial bases of violence.* NATO ASI Series A292. New York: Plenum Press.

Raleigh, M.J., M.T. McGuire, G.L. Brammer, D.B. Pollack, and A. Yuwiler. 1991. Serotonergic mechanisms promote dominance acquisition in adult male vervet monkeys. *Brain Research* 559:181–90.

Raleigh, M.J., M.T. McGuire, G.L. Brammer, and A. Yuwiler. 1984. Social and environmental influences on blood serotonin concentrations in monkeys. *Archives of General Psychiatry* 41:405–10.

Ray, J.J. 1990. The old-fashioned personality. *Human Relations* 43:997–1,015.

Regidor, E., M.E. Calle, P. Navarro, and V. Dominguez. 2003. Trends in the association between average income, poverty and income inequality and life expectancy in men and women in the regions of Spain. *Social Science and Medicine* 56(5):961–71.

Relate/Candis. 1998. *Why we argue.* London: Relate.

Relethford, J.H. 2003. *The human species.* Boston: McGraw-Hill.

Reynolds, V., and G. Luscombe. 1976. Greeting behaviour, displays and rank order in a group of free-ranging chimpanzees. In *The social structure of attention.* Edited by M.R.A. Chance and R. Larsen. New York: Wiley.

Rilling, J.K., D.A. Gutman, T.R. Zeh, G. Pagnoni, G.S. Berns, and C.D. Kilts. 2002. A neural basis for social cooperation. *Neuron* 35:395–405.

Rizzolatti, G., L. Fogassi, and V. Gallese. 2000. Mirror neurons: Intentionality detectors? *International Journal of Psychology* 35(3–4):205.

Rodgers, G.B. 1997. Income and inequality as determinants of mortality: An international cross-section analysis. *Population Studies* 33:343–51.

Rose, G. 1992. *The strategy of preventive medicine.* Oxford: Oxford University Press.

Rose, G., and M.G. Marmot. 1981. Social class and coronary heart disease. *British Heart Journal* 45:13–19.

Ross, N.A., M.C. Wolfson, J.R. Dunn, J.M. Berthelot, G.A. Kaplan, and J.W. Lynch. 2000. Relation between income inequality and mortality in Canada and in the United States: Cross sectional assessment using census data and vital statistics. *British Medical Journal* 320:898–902.

Sable, M.R., and D.S. Wilkinson. 2000. Impact of perceived stress, major life events and pregnancy attitudes on low birth weight. *Family Planning Perspectives* 32(6):288–94.

Sahlins, M. 1974. *Stone age economics.* London: Tavistock.

Sanmartin, C., N.A. Ross, S. Tremblay, M. Wolfson, J.R. Dunn, and J. Lynch. 2003. Labour market income inequality and mortality in North American metropolitan areas. *Journal of Epidemiology and Community Health* 57(10):792–97.

Sapolsky, R.M. 1993. Endocrinology alfresco: Psychoendocrine studies of wild baboons. *Recent Progress in Hormone Research* 48:437–68.

———. 1996. Why stress is bad for your brain. *Science* 273:749–50.

———. 1998. *Why zebras don't get ulcers: A guide to stress, stress-related disease and coping.* 2nd ed. New York: W.H. Freeman.

———. 2001. *A primate's memoir.* London: Jonathan Cape.

Scheff, T.J. 1988. Shame and conformity: the deference-emotion system. *American Sociological Review* 53:395–406.

————. 1990. *Microsociology: Discourse, emotion and social structure.* Chicago: University of Chicago Press.

Scheff, T.J., S.M. Retzinger, and M.T. Ryan. 1989. Crime, violence, and self-esteem: Review and proposals. In *The social importance of self-esteem.* Edited by A.M. Mecca, N.J. Smelser, and J. Vasconcellos. Berkeley: University of California Press.

Schor, J. 1998. *The overspent American: When buying becomes you.* New York: Basic Books.

Schore, A.N. 1998. Early shame experiences and infant brain development. In *Shame: Interpersonal behavior, psychopathology and culture.* Edited by P. Gilbert and B. Andrews. New York: Oxford University Press.

Seeman, T.E. 2000. Health promoting effects of friends and family on health outcomes in older adults. *American Journal of Health Promotion* 14(6):362–70.

Sen, A. 1981. Public action and the quality of life in developing countries. *Oxford Bulletin of Economics and Statistics* 43:287–319.

Shaw, G.B. 1928. *The intelligent woman's guide to socialism and capitalism.* New York: Brentano's.

Shively, C.A., and T.B. Clarkson. 1994. Social status and coronary artery atherosclerosis in female monkeys. *Arteriosclerosis and Thrombosis* 14:721–26.

Sidanius, J., and F. Pratto. 1999. *Social dominance: An intergroup theory of social hierarchy and oppression.* Cambridge: Cambridge University Press.

Smith, A. 1759. *The theory of the moral sentiments.* Reprint. Indianapolis: Liberty Classics, 1952.

Soloman, K. 1981. The masculine gender role and its implications for the life expectancy of older men. *Journal of American Geriatrics Society* 29(7):297–301.

Soobader, M.-J., and F.B. LeClere. 1999. Aggregation and the measurement of income inequality: Effects on morbidity. *Social Science and Medicine* 48(6):733–44.

Stafford, M., M. Bartley, R. Boreham, R. Thomas, R. Wilkinson, and M. Marmot. 2000. Neighbourhood social cohesion and health. In *Social capital and health.* Edited by A. Morgan. London: Health Development Agency.

Stafford, M., M. Bartley, R. Wilkinson, R. Boreham, R. Thomas, A. Sacker, and

M. Marmot. 2003. Measuring the social environment: Social cohesion and material deprivation in English and Scottish neighbourhoods. *Environmental Planning* A 35:1,459–75.

Stam, M.C., R. Koyuncu, E.R. Pelfrene, G. de Backer, and M.D. Kornitzer. 2002. Psychosocial characteristics and coronary risk factors in relation to fibrinogen in a Belgian working population of middle-aged men and women.

Stanistreet, D., A. Scott-Samuel, and M. Bellis. 1999. Income inequality and mortality in England—Is there a threshold effect? *Journal of Public Health Medicine* 21(2):205–7.

Stansfeld, S. 1999. Social support and social cohesion. In *Social determinants of health,* ed. M. Marmot and R.G. Wilkinson. Oxford: Oxford University Press.

Subramanian, S.V., T. Blakely, and I. Kawachi I. 2003. Income inequality as a public health concern: Where do we stand? *Health Services Research* 38(1):153–67.

Subramanian, S.V., I. Delgado, L. Jadue, J. Vega, and I. Kawachi. 2003. Income inequality and health: Multilevel analysis of Chilean communities. *Journal of Epidemiology and Community Health* 57(11):844–48.

Subramanian, S.V., and I. Kawachi. 2004. Income inequality and health: what have we learned so far? *Epidemiologic Reviews* 26:1–14.

Suomi, S.J. 1991. Early stress and adult emotional reactivity in rhesus monkeys. In *The childhood environment and adult disease.* Edited by D. Barker. Chichester: Wiley.

Swift, A. 1995. The sociology of complex equality. In *Pluralism, justice, and equality.* Edited by D. Miller and M. Walzer. Oxford: Oxford University Press.

Tajfel, H., M.G. Billig, R.P. Bundy, and C. Flament. 1971. Social categorization and intergroup behaviour. *European Journal of Social Psychology* 1(2):149–78.

Tarkowska, E., and J. Tarkowski. 1991. Social disintegration in Poland: Civil society or amoral familism? *Telos* 89:103–9.

Teixeira, J.M.A., N.M. Fisk, and V. Glover. 1998. Association between maternal anxiety in pregnancy and increased uterine artery resistance index: Cohort based study. *British Medical Journal* 318:153–57.

Teranishi, H., H. Nakagawa, and M. Marmot. 2001. Social class difference in catch up growth in a national British cohort. *Archives of the Diseases of Childhood* 84:218–21.

Theorell, T. 2004. Democracy at work and its relationship to health. In *Emotional and physiological processes and positive intervention strategies. Research in occupational stress and well-being.* Edited by P.L. Perrewé and D.C. Ganster. Volume 3, 323–27. Amsterdam: Elsevier.

Timio, M., P. Verdecchia, S. Venanzi, S. Gentili, M. Ronconi, B. Francucci, M. Montanari, and E. Bichisao. 1988. Age and blood pressure changes: A 20-year follow up study in 5 in a secluded order. *Hypertension* 12:457–61.

Titmuss, R.M. 1958. War and social policy. In *Essays on the welfare state.* Edited by R.M. Titmuss. London: Unwin.

Tocqueville, A. de. 2000. *Democracy in America.* Translated by Stephen D. Grant. Indianapolis: Hackett.

Trower, P., P. Gilbert, and G. Sherling. 1990. Social anxiety, evolution and self-presentation. In *Handbook of social and evaluation anxiety.* Edited by H. Leitenberg. New York: Plenum Press.

Uslaner, E. 2002. *The moral foundations of trust.* New York: Cambridge University Press.

Vallee, M., W. Mayo, F. Dellu, M. LeMoal, H. Simon, and S. Maccari. 1997. Prenatal stress induces high anxiety and postnatal handling induces low anxiety in adult offspring: Correlation with stress-induced corticosterone secretion. *Journal of Neuroscience* 17:2,626–36.

Veenstra, G. 2002. Social capital and health (plus wealth, income inequality and regional health governance). *Social Science and Medicine* 54(6):849–68.

Venetoulis, J., and C. Cobb. 2004. The Genuine Progress Indicator 1950–2002. Redefining Progress, Oakland, California. Available on the web at: http://www.redefiningprogress.org/publications/gpi_march2004update.pdf.

Verkes, R.J., M.W. Hengeveld, R.C. van der Mast, D. Fekkes, and G.M.J. van Kempen. 1998. Mood correlates with blood serotonin, but not with glucose measures in patients with recurrent suicidal behavior. *Psychiatry Research* 80(3):239–48.

Visconti, K.J., K.J. Saudino, L.A. Rappaport, J.W. Newburger, and D.C.

Bellinger. 2002. Influence of parental stress and social support on the behavioral adjustment of children with transposition of the great arteries. *Developmental and Behavioral Paediatrics* 23(5):314–21.

Vogli, R. de, R. Mistry, R. Gnesotto, and G.A. Cornia. 2004. The relation between income inequality and life expectancy has not disappeared: Evidence from Italy and 22 wealthy nations. *Journal of Epidemiology and Community Health,* forthcoming.

Waal, F.B.M. de, and F. Lanting. 1997. *Bonobo: The forgotten ape.* Berkeley: University of California Press.

Wadhwa, P.D., C. Dunkel-Schetter, A. Chicz-DeMet, M. Porto, and C.A. Sandman. 1996. Prenatal psychosocial factors and the neuroendocrine axis in human pregnancy. *Psychosomatic Medicine* 58:432–46.

Wadsworth, M.E.J. 1984. Early stress and associations with adult health, behaviour and parenting. In *Stress and disability in childhood.* Edited by N.R. Butler and B.D. Corner. Bristol: Wright.

———. 1991. *The imprint of time: Childhood, history and adult life.* Oxford: Clarendon Press.

Wadsworth, M., M. Maclean, D. Kuh, and B. Rodgers. 1990. Children of divorced and separated parents: Summary and review of findings from a long-term follow-up study in the UK. *Family Practice* 7:104–9.

Walberg, P., M. McKee, V. Shkolnikov, L. Chenet, and D.A. Leon. 1998. Economic change, crime, and mortality crisis in Russia: Regional analysis. *British Medical Journal* 317:312–18.

Waldmann, R.J. 1992. Income distribution and infant mortality. *Quarterly Journal of Economics* 107:1,283–1,302.

Waldron, I., M. Nowotarski, M. Freimer, J.P. Henry, et al. 1982. Cross-cultural variation in blood pressure: A quantitative analysis of the relationships of blood pressure to cultural characteristics, salt consumption and body weight. *Social Science and Medicine* 16:419–30.

Watson, P. 1996. Marriage and mortality in Eastern Europe. In *East-West life expectancy gap in Europe: Environmental and non-environmental determinants.* Edited by C. Hertzman, S. Kelly, and M. Bobak. Dordrecht: Kluwer Academic Publishers.

Wennemo, I. 1993. Infant mortality, public policy and inequality—A comparison of 18 industrialised countries 1950–85. *Sociology of Health and Illness* 15:429–46.

Widdowson, E.M. 1951. Mental contentment and physical growth. *Lancet* (June 16):1,316–18.

Wilkinson, R.G. 1973. *Poverty and progress: An ecological model of economic development*. Methuen.

———. 1986. Income and mortality. In *Class and health: Research and longitudinal data*. Edited by R.G. Wilkinson. London: Tavistock.

———. 1992. Income distribution and life expectancy. *British Medical Journal* 304:165–68.

———. 1994. Research note: German income distribution and infant mortality. *Sociology of Health and Illness* 16:260–62.

———. 1996a. *Unhealthy societies: The afflictions of inequality*. London: Routledge.

———. 1996b. Health and civic society in Eastern Europe before 1989. In *East-West life expectancy gap in Europe: Environmental and non-environmental determinants*. Edited by C. Hertzman, S. Kelly, and M. Bobak. Dordrecht: Kluwer Academic Publishers.

———. 1997a. Health inequalities: Relative or absolute material standards? *British Medical Journal* 314:591–95.

———. 1997b. Income, inequality and social cohesion. *American Journal of Public Health* 87:104–6.

Wilkinson, R.G., I. Kawachi, and B. Kennedy. 1998. Mortality, the social environment, crime and violence. *Sociology of Health and Illness* 20(5):578–97.

Williams, R.B., J.C. Barefoot, J.A. Blumenthal, M.J. Helms, L. Luecken, C.F. Pieper, I.C. Siegler, and E.C. Suarez. 1997. Psychosocial correlates of job strain in a sample of working women. *Archives of General Psychiatry* 54(6):543–48.

Williams, R.B., J. Feaganes, J.C. Barefoot. 1995. Hostility and death rates in 10 U.S. cities *Psychosomatic Medicine* 57(1):94.

Williamson, J.B., and U. Boehmer. 1997. Female life expectancy, gender stratification, health status, and level of economic development: A cross-national study of less developed countries. *Social Science and Medicine* 45(2): 305–17.

Wilson, M., and M. Daly. 1997. Life expectancy, economic inequality, homicide, and reproductive timing in Chicago neighbourhoods. *British Medical Journal* 314:1,271–74.

Wolf, N.S., M.E. Gales, E. Shane, and M. Shane. 2001. The developmental trajectory from amodal perception to empathy and communication: The role of mirror neurons in this process. *Psychoanalytic Inquiry* 21(1):94–112.

Woodburn, J. 1982. Egalitarian societies. *Man* 17:431–51.

World Bank. 1993. *The East Asian miracle: Economic growth and public policy.* New York: Oxford University Press.

Yeh, S.R., B.E. Musolf, and D.H. Edwards. 1997. Neuronal adaptations to changes in the social dominance status of crayfish. *Journal of Neuroscience* 17(2):697–708.

Index

Adorno, Theodor, 198, 224–25
affiliative strategies. *See* evolved
   human social strategies
African Americans: group density
   effect and health of, 179; life
   expectancies/death rates, 14–15,
   228–29; and self-esteem, 158–59;
   social inequality and violence,
   150, 155; social status and health,
   14–15, 76, 179, 228–29
agonic social systems, 249–50,
   252
Albania, 117, 206–7
Alexander, Richard D., 183, 258
Anzaldúa, Gloria, 226–27
Aristotle, 184
Asch, S. E., 94
Asian economies, 207–8, 302
aspirational incomes, 173–74,
   312–13
atherosclerosis. *See* heart disease
attachment, 84, 271
Australia, 109, 110
"authoritarian personality,"
   197–98
The Authoritarian Personality (Adorno
   et al.), 198, 224–25

Banfield, E. C., 213, 220
Barker, David, 81–82
Benn, Tony, 248
Beveridge Report (1941), 209
"bicycling reaction," 224–28
biological indicators of psychological
   sensitivity to status, 87–88,
   162–67; blood pressure, 55, 86,
   162, 163–64, 276–77; cortisol
   levels and chronic stress, 74, 83,
   99, 164, 268, 271, 275–77;
   depression and social anxiety, 4–5,
   87–88, 164–66; diseases and
   chronic stress, 79–81, 273, 275–79;
   dopamine levels, 88; fibrinogen
   levels, 163–64; friendship risk
   factor, 88; men and violence,
   166–67; psychobiology evidence,
   87–88; serotonin levels, 87–88,
   165, 280–81; social status risk
   factors, 87–88, 165; stress triggers
   and responses, 162–64; suicides,
   167. *See also* social status; stress,
   chronic; violence and inequality
Bismarck, Otto von, 209, 303
blacks. *See* African Americans
Blau, F. D., 221